CRASH COURSE

Third Edition

Renal and urinary systems

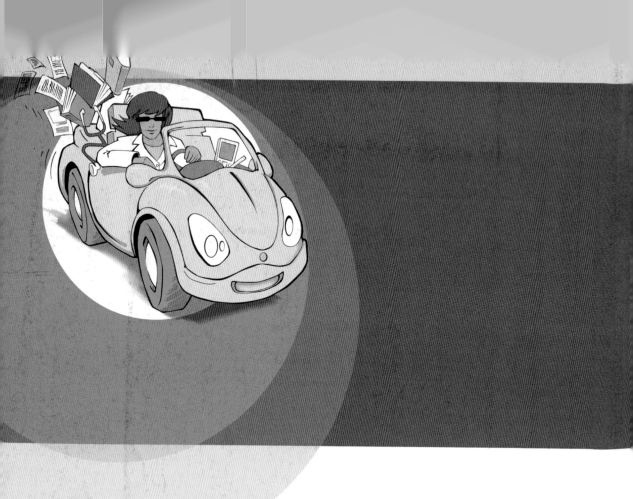

First and second edition authors:

Nisha Mirpuri

Pratiksha Patel

Shreelata Datta

Third Edition

Renal and urinary systems

Series editor
Daniel Horton-Szar
BSc (Hons), MBBS (Hons) MRCGP
Northgate Medical Practice
Canterbury
Kent, UK

Faculty advisor
Kevin Harris
Infection, Immunity and
Inflammation
University of Leicester School
of Medicine
Leicester General Hospital
Leicester, UK

Robert Thomas
Medical student, Medical School, University of Newcastle upon
Tyne, Newcastle upon Tyne, UK

Bethany Stanley
Medical student, University of Leicester School of Medicine,
Leicester, UK

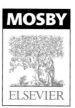

MOSBY

ELSEVIER

Edinburgh • London • New York • Oxford • Philadelphia • St Louis • Sydney • Toronto 2007

MOSBY

ELSEVIER

An imprint of Elsevier Limited

Commissioning Editor	**Alison Taylor**
Development Editor	**Helen Leng**
Project Manager	**Emma Riley**
Text design	**Sarah Russell**
Icon illustrations	**Geo Parkin**
Cover design	**Stewart Larking**
Illustrator	**Cactus**
Illustration Manager	**Merlyn Harvey**

First edition 1998
Second edition 2003
Third edition 2007
  Reprinted 2009

ISBN: 978 0 7234 3428 3

British Library Cataloguing in Publication Data
A catalogue record for this book is available from the British Library

Library of Congress Cataloging in Publication Data
A catalog record for this book is available from the Library of Congress

Note
Neither the publisher nor the authors assume any responsibility for any loss or injury and/or damage to persons or property arising out of or related to any use of the material contained in this book. It is the responsibility of the treating practitioner, relying on independent expertise and knowledge of the patient, to determine the best treatment and method of application for the patient.

ELSEVIER your source for books,
journals and multimedia
in the health sciences
www.elsevierhealth.com

Working together to grow
libraries in developing countries

www.elsevier.com | www.bookaid.org | www.sabre.org

ELSEVIER   BOOK AID
International   Sabre Foundation

The
publisher's
policy is to use
**paper manufactured
from sustainable forests**

Typeset by RDC Publishing Group
Printed in China

Renal and urinary medicine is widely regarded as a complex and difficult area for medical students. This is partly due to the fact that very often the basic principles of the system haven't yet been grasped. With these in place, understanding of the role of the kidneys and their multiple systemic involvement will come much more naturally.

This new edition of *Crash Course: Renal and Urinary Systems* provides students with a thorough overview of renal and urinary medicine. The book is not only designed to help with revision, but to provide a source of current knowledge in this area.

We hope that you find this book useful, and are able to make use of the extensive self-assessment section at the back of the book, with a new extended-matching questions (EMQ) section in keeping with current undergraduate assessment.

Rob Thomas
Bethany Stanley

Diseases of the urinary tract have traditionally been seen as a challenge for medical students. To address this *Crash Course: Renal and Urinary Systems* is written in a way that allows students to develop their knowledge in a balanced and logical way while stimulating them to continue with self-directed learning.

As with all *Crash Course* books, the text is written by a medical student with expert input from a faculty advisor – me – and the series editor. This approach has ensured that the book will provide students with a solid, accurate, user-friendly and relevant overview of the subject. The integrated approach between basic and clinical sciences provides the appropriate theoretical basis for solving the kind of problems that are commonly encountered in clinical practice.

This third edition has been extensively revised, building, where appropriate, on the first and second editions using readers' feedback and suggestions. The text has been updated yet retains its concise and clear style. New images of disease have been added to the already plentiful illustrations and the self-assessment section contains new multiple-choice questions (MCQs), short-answer questions (SAQs) and EMQs.

It's hoped that this book provides students with a useful supplement to their lecture notes and a concise and comprehensive revision aid for testing their knowledge of this fascinating subject.

Dr Kevin Harris
Faculty Advisor

More than a decade has now passed since work began on the first editions of the Crash Course series, and over four years since the publication of the second editions. Medicine never stands still, and the work of keeping this series relevant for today's students is an ongoing process. These third editions build upon the success of the preceding books and incorporate a great deal of new and revised material, keeping the series up to date with the latest medical research and developments in pharmacology and current best practice.

As always, we listen to feedback from the thousands of students who use Crash Course and have made further improvements to the layout and structure of the books. Each chapter now starts with a set of learning objectives, and the self-assessment sections have been enhanced and brought up to date with modern exam formats. We have also worked to integrate points of clinical relevance into the basic medical science material, which will not only add to the interest of the text but will reinforce the principles being described.

Despite fully revising the books, we hold fast to the principles on which we first developed the series: Crash Course will always bring you all the information you need to revise in compact, manageable volumes that integrate basic medical science and clinical practice. The books still maintain the balance between clarity and conciseness, and providing sufficient depth for those aiming at distinction. The authors are medical students and junior doctors who have recent experience of the exams you are now facing, and the accuracy of the material is checked by senior faculty members from across the UK.

I wish you all the best for your future careers!

Dr Dan Horton-Szar
Series Editor

We would like to thank Kevin Harris and Helen Leng for their continuing support and tireless input over the course of working on this edition.

Figure credits
Figures 1.9, 1.10, 3.14 and 3.19 redrawn with kind permission from C J Lote. Principles of renal physiology, 4th edn. Kluwer Academic Publishers, 2000

Figure 2.7 and 2.26 adapted with permission from A Stevens and J Lowe. Human histology, 2nd edn. Mosby, 1997

Figure 8.16 redrawn with permission from L Impey. Obstetrics and gynaecology. Blackwell Science, 1999

I would like to dedicate this book to the memory of my Dad; he never stopped encouraging me.
BS

BASIC MEDICAL SCIENCE OF THE RENAL AND URINARY SYSTEMS

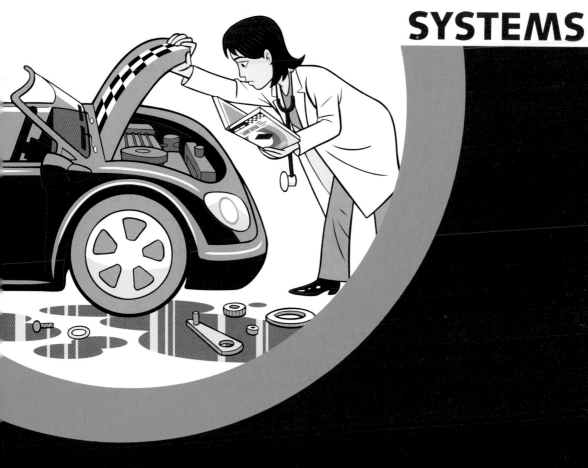

By the end of the chapter you should be able to:

- Describe the location and composition of the kidneys
- Summarize the main functions of the kidney
- Name the different fluid compartments within the body, stating their relative proportions and values
- Distinguish between osmolarity and osmolality, defining the units of measurement for each
- Explain how the following influence the distribution of ions across a semi-permeable membrane:
  - Concentration gradient
  - Electrical gradient
  - Proteins
- Understand the role of the lymphatic system in fluid movement
- Describe the routes by which water and ions enter and leave the body, giving the relevant values
- Outline the difference between the two methods used in the dilution principle
- Discuss why it is important to use high-molecular-weight plasma proteins when measuring plasma volume
- Explain why interstitial fluid must be measured indirectly.

OVERVIEW OF THE KIDNEY AND URINARY TRACT

Structural organization of the kidney and urinary tract

The kidneys lie in the retroperitoneum on the posterior abdominal wall on either side of the vertebral column (T11–L3). The right kidney is displaced by the liver, so it is 12 mm lower than the left kidney. The adult kidney is approximately 11 cm long and 6 cm wide, with a mass of 140 g. Each kidney is composed of two main regions:

- An outer dark brown cortex
- An inner pale medulla and renal pelvis.

The renal pelvis contains the major renal blood vessels and the origins of the ureter. Each kidney consists of 1 million nephrons, which span the cortex and medulla and are bound together by connective tissue containing blood vessels, nerves and lymphatics.

The kidneys form the upper part of the urinary tract. The urine produced by the kidneys is transported to the bladder by two ureters. The lower urinary tract consists of the bladder and the urethra.

Approximately 1–1.5 L of urine is produced by the kidneys each day – the volume and osmolality vary according to fluid intake and fluid loss.

The urinary tract epithelium is impermeable to water and solutes unlike the nephrons in the kidney, so the composition of urine is not altered as it is transported to the bladder. The bladder contents are emptied via the urethra, expulsion from the body being controlled by an external sphincter. Both the upper and the lower urinary tracts are innervated by the autonomic nervous system.

Fig. 1.1 Anatomy of the posterior abdominal wall showing the renal and urinary system. 1, liver; 2, stomach; 3, second part of the duodenum; 4, pancreas.

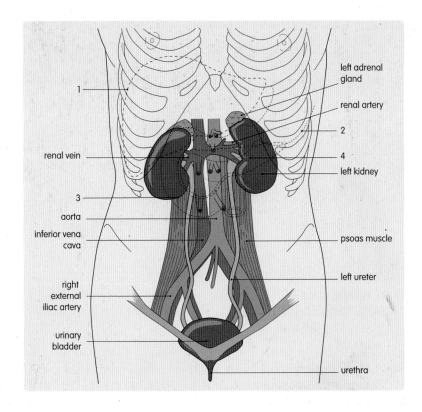

Figure 1.1 shows the anatomy of the kidneys and urinary tract.

Functions of the kidney and the urinary tract

1. **Excretion**: of waste products and drugs – this involves selective reabsorption and excretion of substances as they pass through the nephron.
2. **Regulation**: of body fluid volume and ionic composition. The kidneys have a major role in homeostasis (the maintenance of a constant internal environment) and are also involved in maintaining the acid–base balance.
3. **Endocrine**: the kidneys are involved in the synthesis of renin (which generates angiotensin I from angiotensinogen, and thus has a role in blood pressure and sodium balance), erythropoietin (which controls erythrocyte production) and prostaglandins (involved in vasodilation).
4. **Metabolism**: Vitamin D is metabolized to its active form. The kidney is a major site for the

catabolism of low-molecular-weight proteins including several hormones such as insulin, parathyroid hormone and calcitonin.

FLUID COMPARTMENTS OF THE BODY

Body fluids

Body fluids are divided into:

- Intracellular fluid (ICF), the fluid within cells
- Extracellular fluid (ECF).

ECF is divided into:

- Plasma – ECF within the vascular system, i.e. the non-cellular component of blood.
- Interstitial fluid (ISF) – ECF outside the vascular system (and separated from plasma by the capillary endothelium).
- Transcellular fluid (TCF) – ECF (e.g. synovial fluid, aqueous and vitreous humour,

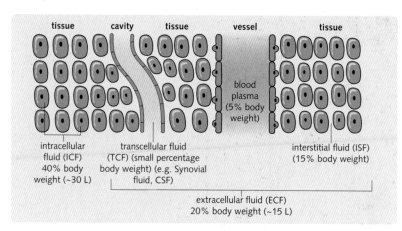

Fig. 1.2 Fluid compartments of the body.

cerebrospinal fluid) separated from plasma by the capillary endothelium and an additional epithelial layer that has specialized functions (Fig. 1.2).

Water is a major component of the human body. Approximately 63% of an adult male and 52% of an adult female is water (i.e. 45 L in a 70 kg male, 36 L in a 70 kg female). This difference is due to the fact that females have a higher proportion of body fat, which has a low water content. One-third of total body water (TBW) is ECF (about 15 L in a 70 kg male) and two-thirds is ICF (about 30 L in a 70 kg male).

Osmolarity and osmolality

Basic concepts

Osmosis is the net passage of a solvent through a semi-permeable membrane from a less concentrated solution to a more concentrated solution. This occurs until both solutions reach the same concentration (equilibrium). The osmotic effect can be measured as an osmotic pressure. This is the pressure at which water is drawn into a solution across a semi-permeable membrane. Thus, the more concentrated the solution (i.e. the higher the solute content), the greater the osmotic pressure. Hydrostatic pressure is the pressure needed to be applied to the region containing the solute to prevent the net entry of water.

Osmolarity is the total solute concentration of a solution – the number of osmotically active particles in solution. The higher the osmolarity, the lower the water concentration.

1 Osmole (Osmol) = 1 mole of solute particles.

Osmolarity versus osmolality

Osmolarity is the molar concentration of solute particles per litre of solution (mOsmol/L). *Osmolality* is the molar concentration of solute particles per kilogram of solvent (water) (mOsmol/kg H_2O). Figure 1.3 illustrates the differences between osmolality and osmolarity.

- Normal body fluid osmolality is between 285 and 295 mOsmol/kg H_2O
- Urine osmolality may vary between 60 and 1400 mOsmol/kg H_2O.

Plasma osmolality can be calculated from sodium ion (Na^{++}), potassium ion (K^{++}), urea, and glucose concentrations using the formula:

Plasma osmolality = 2(Na^{++} + K^{++}) + urea + glucose

Isotonicity and isosmoticity

Changes in the extracellular osmolarity can cause cells to shrink or swell because water will move across the plasma membrane by osmosis into or out of the cells to maintain equilibrium. Therefore, an important function of the kidneys is to regulate the excretion of water in the urine so that the osmolarity of the ECF remains nearly constant despite wide variations in intake or extrarenal losses of salt and water. This prevents damage to the cells from excess swelling and shrinkage:

- If cells are placed in a solution over 295 mOsmol (hypertonic solution), they shrink as water moves out into the solution.

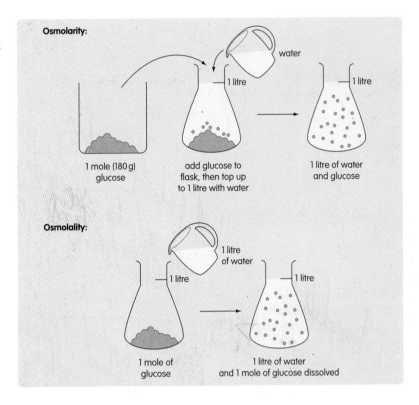

Fig. 1.3 Osmolarity can be described as 1 mole of glucose added to water, and dissolved to make up to 1 L. Osmolality is the addition of 1 L of water to one mole of glucose (adapted from Lote CJ 2000 Principles of renal physiology, 4th edn. Kluwer Academic Publishers, p 4–5).

- If cells are placed in a solution of 285–295m Osmol/kg H_2O (isotonic solution, i.e. 0.9% saline), there is no net movement of water by osmosis and no swelling or shrinkage. This is because an isotonic solution has the same osmolarity as normal body fluid.
- If cells are placed in a solution less than 285 mOsmol (hypotonic solution), they swell as water enters from the solution.

- **Isosmoticity**: this refers to solutions with the same solution concentration per kilogram water (e.g. 0.9% saline and 5% dextrose).
- **Isotonicity**: this refers to solutions that do not cause any change in cell volume (e.g. 285–295 mOsmol/L of non-permeable solute).

Thus, different isotonic solutions are isosmotic, but solutions that are isosmotic to plasma are not necessarily isotonic.

Figure 1.4 shows the changes in the cells brought about by hypertonic, isotonic and hypotonic solutions.

Diffusion of ions across biological membranes

Passive transport

Biological membranes (e.g. cell membranes) are selectively permeable, allowing only small molecules and ions to diffuse through them. The concentration gradient and electrical gradient influence the movement of these molecules into or out of cells.

The rate of diffusion of different molecules depends upon their shape, size, weight and electrical charge. When solutions either side of a membrane contain diffusible ions only, ions move passively from an area of high ionic concentration down the electrical gradient to an area of lower ionic concentration. This occurs until equilibrium is reached, when the ion distribution on either side of the membrane will be as follows:

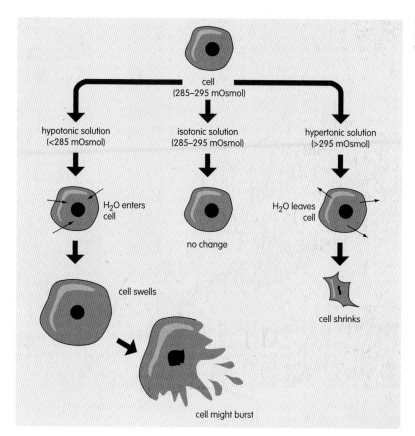

Fig. 1.4 Cell changes induced by hypotonic, isotonic and hypertonic solutions.

Side A (diffusible cations × diffusible anions) =
Side B (diffusible cations × diffusible anions)

The Gibbs–Donnan effect

Proteins are negatively charged molecules, which are so large that they cannot diffuse across membranes. Thus, if proteins are present on one side of the membrane (side A), they act as anions and attract positive ions (cations) from side B. Cations diffuse across the membrane to the more negative side A, and thus maintain electrical neutrality. As a result, side A will not only contain non-diffusible proteins, but also the cations from side B – and therefore will have a greater number of total ions. Consequently, the osmotic pressure on side A will be greater. This encourages the entry of water, unless the osmotic pressure difference is counterbalanced by hydrostatic pressure on side B (Fig. 1.5).

Cell membranes are permeable to:

- Potassium ions (K^+)
- Chloride ions (Cl^-)
- Sodium ions (Na^+).

Active transport

Na^+ permeability is 1/50th K^+ permeability. The primary active transport mechanism uses energy in the form of adenosine triphosphate (ATP) to actively pump Na^+ out of and K^+ into the cells against a concentration gradient. Three Na^+ ions are exchanged for every two K^+ ions. This sodium pump is composed of several proteins and lies within the cell membrane of all cells. Cl^- ions diffuse passively out of the cell across the cell membrane because there is an overall negative charge within the cell. This leads to a higher concentration of Cl^- ions outside the cells. At equilibrium, the cell has a net negative charge (-70 mV).

According to the Gibbs–Donnan effect, there should be more ions inside the cell than outside because of the effects of anionic proteins. This is balanced in biological systems by the sodium pump as Na^+ is effectively non-diffusible.

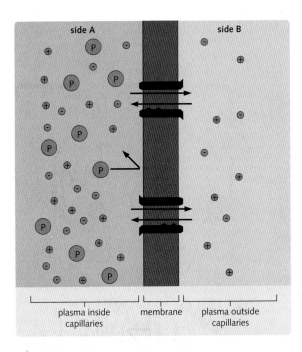

Fig. 1.5 The Gibbs–Donnan effect. +, diffusible cation; – diffusible anion; P, impermeable molecule (e.g. protein).

side A   side B

plasma inside capillaries | membrane | plasma outside capillaries

---

It is very important that water and ions (salt) are kept in balance within the body. Dehydration (loss of water from body tissues) will disrupt these mechanisms. There are three types of dehydration:

- Isosmotic – water loss equals ions loss (diarrhoea, vomiting, burns)
- Hyposmotic – ion loss exceeds water loss (adrenal insufficiency)
- Hyperosmotic – water loss exceeds ion loss (diabetes insipidus, diabetes mellitus).

Fluid movement between body compartments

At any one moment, body fluid compartments have a relatively constant yet dynamic composition. Equilibrium is maintained by the continual transfer of fluid between the different compartments.

Exchange between ECF and ICF

Water diffuses freely across cell membranes so that equilibrium is reached between the ICF and ECF. Any change in the ionic concentration of the ICF or ECF is followed by the movement of water between these compartments.

- Na^+ is the most important extracellular osmotically active ion
- K^+ is the most important intracellular osmotically active ion.

Exchange between plasma and ISF

The capillary endothelium separates plasma (within the circulatory system) from the ISF (outside the circulatory system). Water and ions move between these two compartments – 90% of ions by simple diffusion and 10% by filtration.

Ion filtration between plasma and ISF relies on:

- The arterial end of the capillary, which has a hydrostatic pressure of 32 mmHg, forcing fluid out of the capillary plasma into the ISF.
- Proteins that are too large to cross the capillary endothelial cells, and therefore remain in the plasma, creating a colloid osmotic (or oncotic) pressure (25 mmHg).
- The venous end of the capillary having an osmotic pressure of 25 mmHg. This is greater than the hydrostatic pressure (12 mmHg), causing fluid to move out of the ISF and re-enter the capillary plasma.

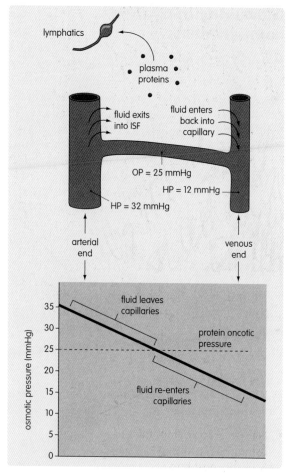

Fig. 1.6 Starling forces – factors involved in fluid exchange between the plasma and ISF across a capillary wall. HP, hydrostatic pressure; OP, oncotic pressure. *Note*: HP decreases from the arterial to the venous end of the capillary; OP is constant throughout.

Water diffusion is controlled by two forces:

- Hydrostatic pressure (within the vascular system only)
- Osmotic pressure (from plasma proteins).

Albumin is the main plasma protein responsible for maintaining osmotic pressure and plasma volume. Abnormally low levels may result in a loss of oncotic pressure in the blood vessels. This results in the retention of fluid in the ISF, causing swelling of the tissue, a clinical sign called oedema.

Exchange between interstitial fluid and lymphatic vessels

Plasma proteins and fluid lost from the vascular system are filtered into the ISF and taken up by the lymphatic system. The lymphatic system is composed of a network of lymphatic capillaries in all organs and tissues, which eventually drain into the venous system via the thoracic duct in the neck. These lymphatic capillaries are very permeable to protein and thus return both the fluid and plasma proteins to the circulatory system.

The ionic composition of the fluid compartments is shown in Figure 1.7.

The movement of fluid across a capillary wall between the plasma and ISF is illustrated in Figure 1.6.

Hydrostatic pressure depends upon:

- Arteriole blood pressure
- Arteriole resistance (which determines the extent to which blood pressure is transferred to the capillary)
- Venous blood pressure.

Osmotic pressure (25 mmHg) is produced by plasma proteins (17 mmHg – oncotic pressure) and the imbalance of ions – there are more ions (e.g. Na^+) within the capillary than outside. This is due to the presence of negatively charged proteins and the Gibbs–Donnan effect.

Fig. 1.7 Composition of the body fluid compartments			
Component	Plasma	ECF	ICF*
Na^+ (mmol/L)	142	145	12
K^+ (mmol/L)	4	4.1	150
Cl^- (mmol/L)	103	113	4
HCO_3^- (mmol/L)	25	27	12
proteins (g/L)	60	0	25
osmolality (mOsm/kg H_2O)	280	280	280
compartment volume (L)	3.0	12.0	30

*ICF compartment is not the same throughout the body; it varies with different types of cell

Fig. 1.8 Distribution of daily water ingestion and losses

Water intake (mL)		Water output (mL)	
drink	1500	lungs	400
food	500	skin	400
metabolism	400	faeces	100
		urine	1500
total	2400	total	2400

Fluid and ion movement between the body and the external environment

There is a continuous exchange of body fluids with the external environment, but there must be a balance between intake and output, as body weight is consistent from day to day.

Daily water intake and output are shown in Figure 1.8. Water loss from the lungs varies with the climate (e.g. in very dry climates over 400 mL per day is lost). Insensible losses are those due to evaporation of water from the skin (i.e. not sweat). Sweating ('sensible perspiration') is an additional loss, which acts as a homeostatic mechanism to maintain constant body temperature. Urinary loss can be adjusted according to the needs of the body and the water intake. The amount of water lost in defaecation can also vary, and is increased greatly in diarrhoea. Daily water intake can fluctuate considerably and can be altered according to need (i.e. thirst mechanism). Water derived from metabolism is the result of oxidation of food. Despite these variations, the body's ionic concentration is maintained within the normal range by the kidney's homeostatic mechanisms, which include control of tubular reabsorption of filtered Na^+– and to a lesser extent K^+ – as well as regulating water reabsorption.

Whereas water intake can be controlled, normally, the minimum water loss from urine, lungs, skin and faeces cannot fall below 1200 mL/day. Thus, if there is no water intake, dehydration occurs, eventually resulting in death within a few days.

Measuring body fluid compartments

Dilution principle

The dilution principle is used to measure fluid volume if fluids cannot be directly measured or extracted from the container or compartment holding them. This allows measuring in situ. A substance that will mix completely and uniformly in the fluid compartment is used to allow all of the volume present to be measured, e.g. a dye. Allowances must be made for the excretion and metabolism of the selected indicator by the body.

$$V_D = \frac{(Q_A - Q_H)}{C}$$

Where V_D = volume of distribution; Q_A = quantity administered; Q_H = quantity metabolized after 10 h; C = concentration.

Two methods are used:
- Single injection method
- Constant infusion method.

Single injection method

This is used for test substances with a slow rate of excretion from the compartment being measured and is carried out as follows:

1. A known amount of test substance is injected intravenously
2. Plasma concentration is determined at intervals
3. A graph (log concentration against time scale) is plotted (Fig. 1.9)
4. The linear portion is extrapolated back to the start (i.e. time 0) – this gives the concentration of substance assuming it had distributed evenly and instantly.

Using this method:

$$\text{Compartment volume} = \frac{\text{Amount injected}}{\text{Concentration at zero time}}$$

Constant infusion method

This is used for test substances that are excreted rapidly and is carried out as follows:

1. A loading dose of the test substance is injected intravenously
2. The test substance is infused at a rate to match the excretion rate
3. Plasma concentration is measured at intervals

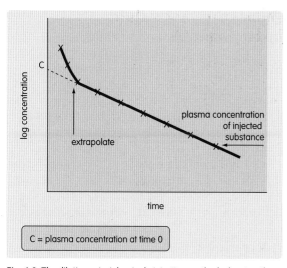

Fig. 1.9 The dilution principle: single injection method, showing the plasma concentration of an injected substance.

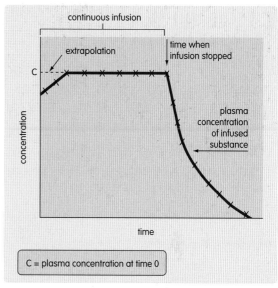

Fig. 1.10 The dilution principle: constant infusion method, showing the plasma concentration of an infused substance.

4. When the substance comes to equilibrium, the plasma concentration is constant (Fig. 1.10)
5. The infusion is stopped and urine collected until all the test substance has been excreted. Using this method:

Amount excreted = Amount present in the body at the time the infusion was stopped

and:

$$\text{Compartment volume (L)} = \frac{\text{Amount excreted (mg)}}{\text{Plasma concentration (mg/L)}}$$

Measurement of plasma volume, red cell volume and blood volume

Plasma volume, blood volume and red cell volume are measured as follows:

• **Plasma volume**: is measured using the dilution principle. The test substance needs to remain within the vascular system (e.g. high-molecular-weight substance). Radio-iodinated human serum albumin and Evans Blue dye are commonly used.

Normal plasma volume = 3 L.

• **Blood volume**: is derived from the kidney plasma volume and the haematocrit (% of red blood cells in total blood volume). For example, if the haematocrit is 45%, the plasma volume is 55% of blood volume (measure plasma volume as above and blood volume = plasma volume × 100/55).

Normal blood volume = 5 L.

• **Red cell volume**: can be derived from plasma volume and haematocrit or measured by direct dilution, using radiolabelled red blood cells.

Measurement of extracellular fluid

As ECF is made up of several compartments (plasma, ISF and TCF), it is difficult to measure accurately. A substance that will diffuse quickly across the endothelial barriers into the ISF, but not into the cells, is required. Substances used include:

• Inulin (can be excluded from bone and cartilage)
• Mannitol
• Thiosulphate (most commonly used)
• Radiosulphate
• Thiocyanate
• Radiochloride or radiosodium (these substances cannot be completely excluded from cells).

A known amount of the selected indicator is injected intravenously and the ECF volume is calculated using the dilution principle. It is difficult to measure the TCF because it is separated from the capillaries by another membrane in addition to the capillary membrane.

Normal ECF volume = 15 L.

Measurement of interstitial fluid

The ISF cannot be measured directly, and it is calculated using the following equation:

ISF (12 L) = ECF (15 L) − plasma volume (3 L)

Measurement of total body water

Isotopes of water are used as markers (deuterium oxide or tritiated water) to measure TBW. The normal value in a 70 kg man is 63% (i.e. 45 L) and in a 70 kg woman, 52% (36 L), being lower in women because of their greater proportion of body fat.

Measurement of transcellular fluid

As this compartment is separated from the rest of the ECF by a membrane, the substances used to measure the ECF do not cross into this compartment. Thus TCF is included in the TBW, but excluded from the ECF:

TBW = ECF + ICF + TCF

There is a large turnover – about 20 L/day in the gastrointestinal tract. Figure 1.11 summarizes the methods used to measure the different fluid volumes.

Fig. 1.11 Summary of fluid compartments and their measurement in an individual weighing 70 kg

Fluid volume	Normal volume	Method of measurement
plasma volume	3 L	radio-iodinated human serum albumin or Evans blue dye
blood volume	5 L	determined from the haematocrit
red cell volume	2 L	• measured from plasma volume and haematocrit • direct dilution
extracellular fluid (ECF)	15 L	indirect measurement using an injected substance (e.g. inulin)
intracellular fluid	28 L	ICF = TBW − ECF − TCF
interstitial fluid (ISF)	12 L	calculated from ECF and plasma volume
total body water (TBW)	63% of total mass (men) 53% of total mass (women)	isotopes of water are used as markers
transcellular fluid (TCF)	20 L/day turnover in the gut	TCF = TBW − ECF − ICF

Organization of the kidneys

Objectives

By the end of the chapter you should be able to:

- Describe the anatomical relations of the right and left kidneys
- Describe the structure of the five anatomical regions of the nephron
- Name the two different types of nephron, and give three ways in which they differ
- List four hormones that act on the kidney and four that are produced by the kidney
- Discuss how the kidney is involved in vitamin D metabolism
- Describe the structure of the glomerular filter
- Explain how the molecular size and charge of particles affects filtration
- Define reabsorption, secretion and excretion
- Describe the difference between primary and secondary active transport
- Outline sodium handling by the proximal tubule
- Using a graph, explain how glucose reabsorption in the proximal tubule is 'T_m limited'
- Name two other substances reabsorbed in the proximal tubule whose T_m is also limited
- Discuss the reabsorption of HCO_3^- in the proximal tubule
- Summarize the countercurrent mechanism of the loop of Henle
- Explain how antidiuretic hormone (ADH) affects urine concentration.

DEVELOPMENT OF THE KIDNEYS

The kidneys pass through three embryological developmental stages (Fig. 2.1):

1. **Pronephros:** is the most primitive system, developing in the cervical region of the embryo during the fourth week of gestation. It is non-functional and regresses soon after its formation, leaving behind a nephritic duct.
2. **Mesonephros:** develops in the lumbar region and functions for a short period. It consists of excretory tubules with their own collecting ducts known as mesonephric ducts. These drain into the nephritic ducts.
3. **Metanephros:** develops in the sacral region at approximately 5 weeks' gestation and eventually forms the final adult kidneys. It becomes functional in the latter half of the pregnancy.

The functional unit of the kidney – the nephron – develops from the fusion of the:

- **Metanephric blastema**, which develops from the nephrogenic cord (part of the intermediate mesoderm). This forms the nephron tubular system from the glomerulus to the distal tubule.

- **Ureteric bud**, which is an outgrowth of the mesonephric duct. This eventually dilates and splits to form the renal pelvis, calyces and collecting tubules.

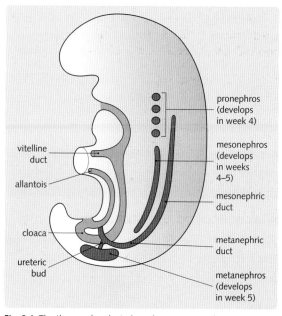

Fig. 2.1 The three embryological renal stages: pronephros, mesonephros and metanephros.

The mesonephric tissue forms a cap over the ureteric bud (ampulla), which grows towards the metanephric blastoma, dilates and divides repeatedly. This eventually forms the pelvis, the major and minor calyces and the collecting ducts of the kidneys. The ampulla differentiates into the nephron once fusion with the metanephric blastema is complete. A solid clump of cells near the differentiating ampulla is converted into a vesicle and fuses with the ampulla to eventually become a web of capillaries known as the glomerulus.

The metanephros initially relies on the pelvic branches of the aorta for its blood supply. Later on, the kidney ascends to the lumbar region and its primary blood supply is from the renal arteries, which branch from the aorta. Finally, the hilum of the kidney rotates from its anterior position to rest medially.

The ureters develop from the part of the ureteric bud between the pelvis and the vesicourethral canal (this develops from part of the hindgut known as the cloaca). They drain into the mesonephric ducts and the urogenital sinus. The urinary bladder develops from the mesoderm, and its epithelium is derived from both the mesoderm (the mesonephric ducts) and the endoderm (vesicourethral canal). This is summarized in Figure 2.2.

The kidneys and the urinary system both develop from the intermediate mesoderm (at the back of the fetal abdominal cavity).

Sometimes a kidney may fail to ascend, remaining located in the pelvis. This is known as a **pelvic kidney**. At other times, the kidneys may be pushed so close together during their ascent that they fuse at the lower poles forming a **horseshoe kidney**.

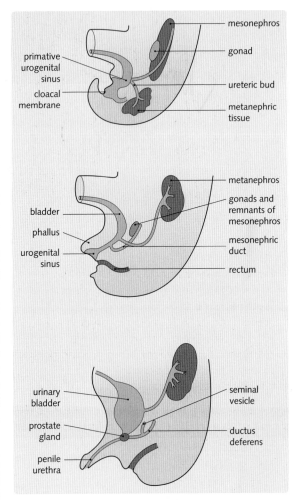

Fig. 2.2 Development of the kidneys, ureters and bladder.

GENERAL ORGANIZATION OF THE KIDNEYS

Macroscopic organization

The anatomy of the kidneys is shown in Figure 2.3. The relations of the kidneys are as follows:

- **Anterior** (Fig. 2.4): to the right kidney – liver, second part of the duodenum and the colon; to the left kidney – stomach, pancreas, spleen, jejunum and descending colon.

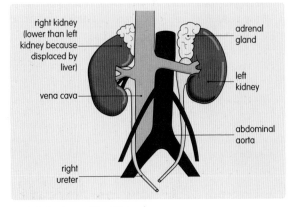

Fig. 2.3 Anatomy of the kidneys.

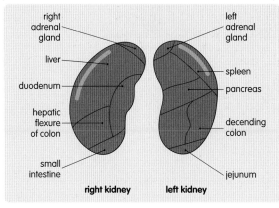

Fig. 2.4 Anterior relations of the right and left kidneys.

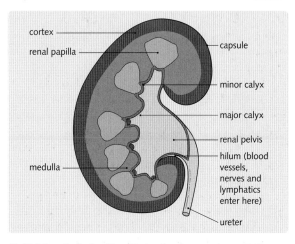

Fig. 2.5 Longitudinal section showing the macroscopic organization of the kidney.

- **Posterior**: diaphragm, quadratus lumborum, psoas, 12th rib and three nerves (subcostal, iliohypogastric and ilioinguinal).
- **Medial**: hilum (a deep fissure containing the renal vessels, nerves, lymphatics and the renal pelvis); to the left kidney – aorta; to the right kidney – inferior vena cava.
- **Superior**: adrenal gland.

The kidneys lie in a fatty cushion (perinephric fat) contained within the renal fascia. They have three capsular layers:

1. Fascial (renal fascia)
2. Fatty (perinephric fascia)
3. True (fibrous capsule).

Morphology and internal structure

Within the kidney, the ureter continues as the renal pelvis, which lies in a deep fissure called the hilum. The outer border of the renal pelvis divides into two or three major divisions (calyces). These subdivide into a number of minor calyces and are each indented by a papilla of renal tissue called the renal pyramid. It is here that the collecting tubules empty the urine. Along with the renal pelvis, the renal artery, vein, nerve and lymphatics all enter the medial border of the kidney at the hilum (Fig. 2.5).

The kidney is divided into two main layers:

1. Outer renal cortex (dark)
2. Inner renal medulla (paler).

The glomeruli in the cortex give it a granular appearance on histological examination.

The blood supply to the kidneys is from the right and left renal arteries, which branch directly off the abdominal aorta at the level of L1–2. The renal veins drain from the kidneys directly into the vena cava. Lymphatics drain to the para-aortic lymph nodes. The kidney is innervated by sympathetic fibres, mainly from the coeliac plexus.

Nephrons

Each kidney has approximately 1 million nephrons. The nephron (Fig. 2.6) is the functional unit of the kidney and consists of:

- A renal corpuscle (Bowman's capsule and the glomerulus)
- Tubule (proximal tubule, loop of Henle, distal tubule and collecting duct).

There are two types of nephron, depending on the length of the loop of Henle:

- **Cortical nephrons**: these have renal corpuscles in the outer part of the cortex, with a correspondingly short loop of Henle.
- **Juxtamedullary nephrons**: these have larger renal corpuscles in the inner third of the cortex, with long loops of Henle extending into the medulla.

In the human kidney, 85% of the nephrons are cortical nephrons and the remaining 15% are juxtamedullary nephrons.

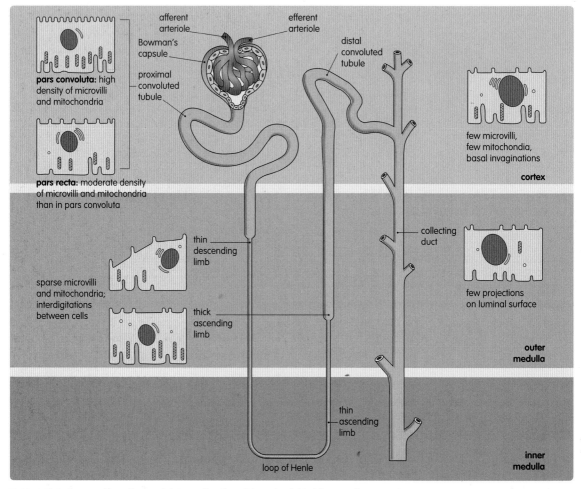

pars convoluta: high density of microvilli and mitochondria

pars recta: moderate density of microvilli and mitochondria than in pars convoluta

sparse microvilli and mitochondria; interdigitations between cells

afferent arteriole

efferent arteriole

Bowman's capsule

proximal convoluted tubule

distal convoluted tubule

thin descending limb

thick ascending limb

thin ascending limb

loop of Henle

collecting duct

few microvilli, few mitochondia, basal invaginations

cortex

few projections on luminal surface

outer medulla

inner medulla

Fig. 2.6 The structure of a nephron and the main histological features of the different cell types within it.

Glomerulus

The glomerulus is formed by the invagination of a ball of capillaries into the Bowman's capsule, which is the blind end of a nephron. It has a diameter of approximately 200 μm.

The function of the glomerulus is to produce a protein-free filtrate from the blood in the glomerular capillaries. The capillaries are supplied by the afferent arterioles and drained by the efferent arterioles. The filtration membrane of the renal corpuscle is made up of three layers and is fundamental to kidney function.

Proximal tubule

The proximal tubule continues from the renal corpuscle. It is 15 mm long and 55 μm in diameter.

Its wall is composed of a single layer of cuboidal cells, which interdigitate extensively and are connected by tight junctions at their luminal surfaces. The luminal edge of each cell is made up of millions of microvilli, forming a dense brush border that increases the surface area available for absorption of tubular filtrate. At the base of each cell there are infoldings of the cell membrane (see Fig. 2.6). The extracellular space between the cells is known as the lateral intercellular space.

The structure of the proximal tubule varies along its length:

- The first part is convoluted (pars convoluta) and cells have an increased density of microvilli and a greater number of mitochondria than cells in the second straight part. This suggests a role in transport of substances across the lumen and the filtrate.

- The second straight part (pars recta) leads on to the first part of the loop of Henle (the thin descending limb).

Loop of Henle

The loop of Henle consists of a single layer of flattened squamous cells, which form a thin-walled, hairpin-shaped tube. The cells of the thin descending segment interdigitate sparingly and have few mitochondria and microvilli on the luminal surface (see Fig. 2.6). This segment ends at the tip of the hairpin loop.

The thin ascending segment is 2 mm long and $20\,\mu m$ in diameter. Its structure is similar to the preceding part of the tubule (the pars recta), except that the cells have extensive interdigitations. This might have a role in the active transport and permeability properties of the cells. There is an abrupt transition between the thin and thick ascending segments and the level of this depends on the length of the loop.

The thick ascending segment is 12 mm in length and consists of a single layer of columnar cells. The luminal membrane is invaginated to form many projections, although there is no brush border and there are few infoldings of the basal membrane.

Distal tubule

The distal convoluted tubule is the continuation of the loop of Henle into the cortex, ending in the collecting ducts. The cells have very few microvilli, no brush border and basal infoldings surrounding mitochondria that gradually decrease towards the collecting ducts (see Fig. 2.6). The basal membranes have Na^+/K^+ ATPase pump activity (see p. 26).

Different cell types in this part of the tubule include:

- **Principal cells (P cells)**: these contain few mitochondria and respond to antidiuretic hormone (ADH) – also known as vasopressin.
- **Intercalated cells (I cells)**: these contain lots of mitochondria and secrete hydrogen ions (H^+).

Collecting ducts

The cortical collecting ducts are 20 mm long. They are lined with cuboidal cells that have a few projections on the luminal surface (see Fig. 2.6).

The ducts pass through the renal cortex and medulla and, at the apices of the renal pyramids, drain the urine into the renal pelvis. The renal pelvis is lined by transitional epithelium.

In the cortex each collecting duct drains approximately six distal tubules. In the medulla the collecting ducts join together in pairs to form ducts of Bellini and from here drain into the renal calyx.

Renal function and urine formation depends on three basic processes:

1. Glomerular filtration
2. Tubular reabsorption
3. Tubular secretion.

Blood supply and vascular structure

The kidneys receive 20–25% of the total cardiac output (1.2 L/min) via the right and left renal arteries. These branch to form interlobar arteries, which further divide to form the arcuate arteries (located at the junction between the cortex and medulla). The interlobular arteries arise at 90 degrees to the arcuate arteries through the cortex, dividing to form the afferent arterioles. These form glomerular capillary networks and come together to form the efferent arterioles.

The efferent arterioles drain blood from the glomerular capillaries and act as portal vessels (i.e. carry blood from one capillary network to another).

- In the outer two-thirds of the cortex the efferent arterioles form a network of peritubular capillaries that supplies all cortical parts of the nephron.
- In the inner third of the cortex the efferent arterioles follow a hairpin course to form a capillary network surrounding the loops of Henle and the collecting ducts down into the medulla. These vessels are known as the vasa recta.

The vasa recta and the peritubular capillaries drain into the left and right renal veins and then into the inferior vena cava. The microcirculation of the kidney is illustrated in Fig. 2.7.

The intricate structure and complex nature of the renal blood supply make it very susceptible to damage. The glomerulus may be damaged by high blood pressure and high blood sugar levels in diabetes mellitus. Inflammatory conditions such as glomerulonephritis also lead to disruption of the glomerular capillary filter which results in the presence of blood and protein in the urine (haematuria and proteinuria, respectively).

Function of the renal blood supply

The high rate of blood flow through the kidney is very important in maintaining the homeostatic functions of the kidney. The blood flow through the kidney determines the filtration rate. The oxygen consumption of the kidney is 18 mL/min – 50% of which is involved in Na^+ reabsorption in the tubules. The vasa recta helps deliver oxygen and nutrients to the nephron segments, and allows the return of reabsorbed substances into the circulation.

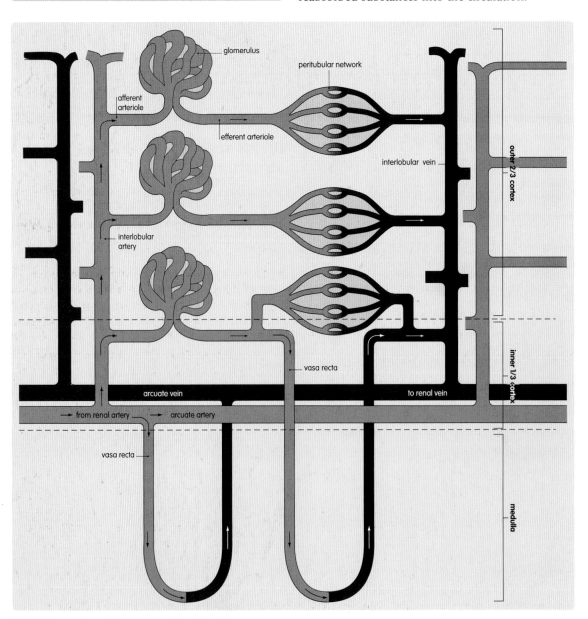

Fig. 2.7 Organization of the blood circulation of the kidney.

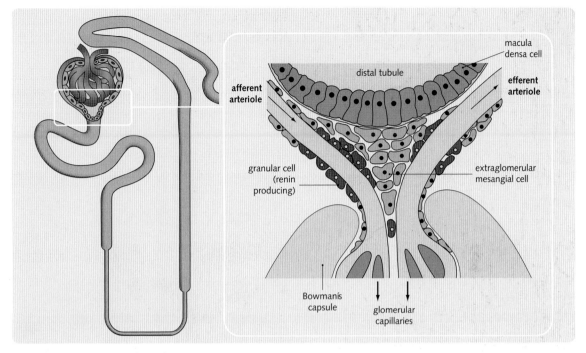

Fig. 2.8 Histology of the juxtaglomerular apparatus.

Although there is substantial blood flow, the arteriovenous oxygen difference is only about 15 mL/L, compared with 62 mL/L in the brain and 114 mL/L in the heart. This means that the oxygen extraction in the kidney is not as efficient as in other organs as a result of shunting of blood in the vasa recta through its hairpin structure.

Juxtaglomerular apparatus

The juxtaglomerular apparatus (JGA) (Fig. 2.8) is located where the thick ascending loop of Henle passes back up into the cortex and lies adjacent to the renal corpuscle and arterioles of its own nephron. It is the area of distal tubule associated with arterioles. The tunica media in the wall of the afferent arteriole contains an area of specialized thickened cells (granular cells), which secrete renin. The epithelium of the distal tubule forms specialized macula densa cells that respond to changes in the composition of the tubular fluid, especially the concentration of sodium ions ([Na^+]) in the filtrate. Extraglomerular mesangial cells (Goormaghtigh cells) or lacis cells are found outside the glomerulus, in association with the glomerular apparatus. They are contractile cells identical to the mesangial cells.

Hormones produced by the kidney

Renin

Renin is a protein that acts on angiotensinogen to form angiotensin I, which in turn is converted to angiotensin II. Angiotensin II is a potent vasoconstrictor affecting blood pressure, tubular reabsorption of Na^+, and aldosterone secretion from the adrenal glands. Renin release is stimulated by sympathetic stimulation of the granular cells or a decrease in filtrate Na^+ concentration. The latter can occur following a fall in plasma volume, vasodilation of the afferent arterioles and renal ischaemia.

Erythropoietin

The kidney is the major source (85%) of erythropoietin (EPO) production in the adult; in fetal life the liver also produces EPO. It is produced by the peritubular interstitium and the cells of the inner cortex. EPO-sensitive cells are the erythrocyte stem cells found in the bone marrow and the effect of the hormone is to increase the production of erythrocytes, resulting in an increase in the oxygen-carrying capacity of the blood. The half-life of EPO is 5 h.

Clinical use of EPO

Hypoxia, anaemia and renal ischaemia all stimulate EPO synthesis (this is a prostaglandin-mediated response). Increased secretion can be seen in polycystic kidney disease and renal cell carcinoma, resulting in polycythaemia. Patients with chronic renal failure often have inappropriately low EPO secretion, resulting in normochromic normocytic anaemia. Administration of recombinant EPO (either intravenous or subcutaneous) will correct the anaemia of chronic renal failure.

Vitamin D

Vitamin D is a steroid hormone that is found in foods and is also synthesized in the skin from 7-dehydrocholesterol in the presence of sunlight. This naturally occurring vitamin D (cholecalciferol) is hydroxylated in the liver to form 25-hydroxy-cholecalciferol ($25(OH)D_3$). It is further hydroxylated in the proximal tubules under the influence of the enzyme 1a-hydroxylase to form the active metabolite 1,25-dihydroxycholecalciferol ($1,25(OH)_2D_3$). Production of $1,25(OH)_2D_3$ is regulated by parathyroid hormone (PTH), phosphate, and by negative feedback. Active vitamin D is essential for the mineralization of bones and promotes the absorption of calcium ions (Ca^{2+}) and phosphate from the gut.

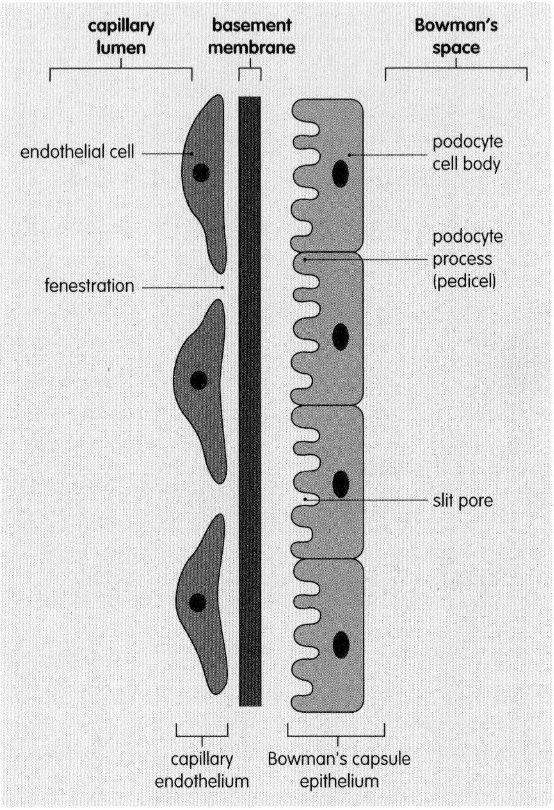

Fig. 2.9 Microscopic organization of the glomerular capillary membrane.

GLOMERULAR STRUCTURE AND FUNCTION

Structure of the glomerular filter

The first stage of urine production is the filtration of plasma through the glomerular capillary wall into the Bowman's capsule. The composition of the plasma ultrafiltrate depends on the filtration barrier, which has three layers (Fig. 2.9):

1. The endothelial cells of the glomerular capillary
2. A basement membrane
3. The epithelial cells of Bowman's capsule.

Endothelial cells

The endothelial cells lining the glomerular capillaries are thin and flat with a large nucleus. The cells are perforated by numerous fenestrae (pores), which have a diameter of 60 nm. This allows plasma components to cross the vessel wall, but not blood cells or platelets.

Basement membrane

The basement membrane is a continuous layer of connective tissue and glycoproteins. It is a non-cellular structure that prevents any large molecules from being filtered.

Epithelial lining

The epithelial lining of Bowman's capsule consists of a single layer of cells (podocytes), which rest on the basement membrane. The podocytes have large extensions or trabeculae, which extend out from the cell body and are embedded in the basement membrane surrounding a capillary. Small processes called pedicels extend out from the trabeculae and inter-digitate extensively with the pedicels of adjacent trabeculae. This leads to the formation of slit pores, which control the movement of substances through the final layer of the filter. The podocytes have a well-developed Golgi apparatus, used to produce and maintain the glomerular basement membrane.

Podocytes can also be involved in phagocytosis of macromolecules (Figs 2.9 and 2.10).

Mesangium

The mesangium is also part of the renal corpuscle and consists of two components:

1. Mesangial cells
2. Mesangial matrix.

The mesangial cells surround the glomerular capillaries and have a function similar to monocytes. They provide structural support for the capillaries, exhibit phagocytic activity, secrete extracellular matrix, and secrete prostaglandins. The cells are contractile, which helps regulate blood flow through the glomerular capillaries (Fig. 2.11).

Process of glomerular filtration

Filtration of macromolecules depends on molecular weight, shape and electrical charge. It is a passive process that involves the flow of a solvent through a filter; any molecules that are small enough to pass through the filter form the filtrate. The glomerular filter allows only low-molecular-weight substances in plasma to pass through it, forming the glomerular ultrafiltrate.

Glomerular filtration rate

The glomerular filtration rate (GFR) is the amount of filtrate that is produced from the blood flowing through the glomerulus per unit time.

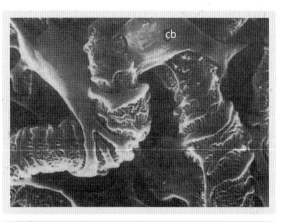

A

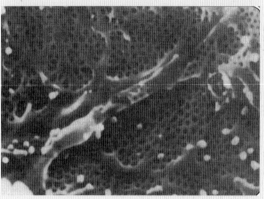

B

Fig. 2.10 Electron micrographs showing the arrangement of podocytes and glomerular capillaries as seen from Bowman's capsule. (A) Processes of podocytes run from the cell body (cb) towards the capillaries where they ultimately split into foot processes (pedicels). (B) Inner surface of a glomerular capillary (from Koeppen BM, Stanton B 1996 Renal physiology, 2nd edn. Mosby Year Book).

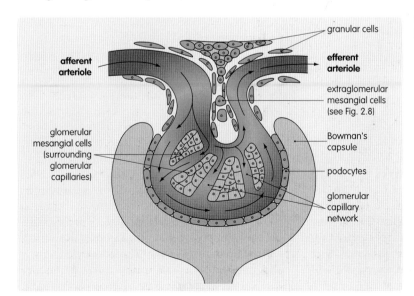

Fig. 2.11 Location of extraglomerular and glomerular mesangial cells.

granular cells

afferent arteriole

efferent arteriole

extraglomerular mesangial cells (see Fig. 2.8)

glomerular mesangial cells (surrounding glomerular capillaries)

Bowman's capsule

podocytes

glomerular capillary network

Fig. 2.12 Forces involved in tissue fluid formation in a non-renal (A) and a renal (B) vascular bed (see text for detailed explanation).

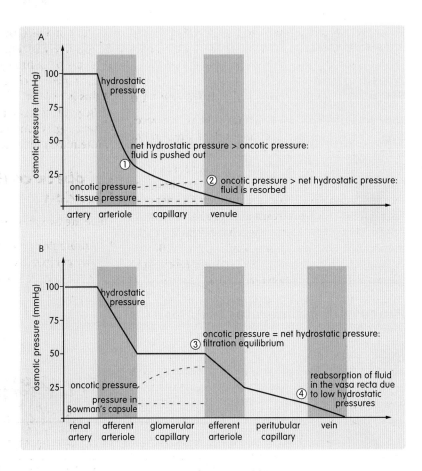

- Normal GFR is 90–120 mL/min/1.73 m² (i.e. corrected for body surface area)
- The total amount filtered is 180 L/day.

The glomerular filtrate normally:

- Contains no blood cells or platelets
- Contains virtually no protein
- Is composed mostly of organic solutes with a low molecular weight and inorganic ions.

Molecular size

Molecular weight is the main factor in determining whether a substance is filtered or remains in the capillaries. The maximum molecular weight of substances able to pass through the filter is 70 kDa. Any molecule with a molecular weight of less than 70 kDa passes freely through the filter (e.g. glucose, amino acids, Na^+, urea, K^+). The shape and electro-chemical charge of macromolecules also affect filter-ability. All three layers of the filter are coated with anions and these repel negatively charged macro-

molecules such as albumin. Smaller, positively charged molecules pass through the filtration barriers relatively easily, unless they are protein bound.

Forces governing tissue fluid formation

The movement of fluid between plasma and tissue fluid is determined by Starling's forces (Fig. 2.12):

- Hydrostatic pressure (due to water)
- Colloid osmotic (oncotic) pressure (due to protein)

Changes in these forces alter the GFR.

The following factors affect tissue fluid formation:

- At the arteriole end of the capillary, hydrostatic pressure is greater than colloid oncotic pressure as a result of resistance to flow due to the narrowing of the vessel, and fluid is forced out of the capillary – point 1 in Figure 2.12A.
- As the fluid moves out of capillaries via the highly permeable wall, oncotic pressure increases and the pressure forces are reversed

(most apparent at the venous end of the capillary) so there is net movement of fluid back into the capillaries – point 2 in Figure 2.12A.

Forces governing glomerular filtration rate

GFR is also driven by Starling's forces. However, in the renal vascular bed the surface area of the glomerular capillaries is much larger than that of normal capillary beds, so there is less resistance to flow. The hydrostatic pressure falls less along the length of the capillary because the efferent arterioles, which act as secondary resistance vessels, maintain a constant pressure along the entire length of the glomerular capillary – point 3 in Figure 2.12B.

Tissue fluid in a vascular bed is the equivalent of glomerular filtrate in Bowman's space, produced as a result of the glomerular capillary hydrostatic pressure (50 mmHg). This is opposed by the hydrostatic pressure in Bowman's capsule (12 mmHg) and the colloid oncotic pressure (25 mmHg) within the capillary. When these forces are equal the filtration equilibrium is reached, with very little fluid movement after this.

Fluid is reabsorbed into the peritubular capillaries – point 4 in Figure 2.12B – as a result of high colloid oncotic pressure (35 mmHg) and low hydrostatic pressure. This reabsorption causes a fall in colloid oncotic pressure as plasma proteins become diluted.

The pressures controlling glomerular filtration into Bowman's capsule are illustrated in Figure 2.13 and the composition of the glomerular filtrate is shown in Figure 2.14.

Albumin has a molecular weight of 69 kDa and is a negatively charged protein. Only very tiny amounts pass through the glomerular filter because of the repelling effect of its negative charge, and all of this is reabsorbed in the proximal tubule. A total of 30 g of protein a day enters the renal lymph vessels. Significant amounts of protein in the urine (proteinuria) indicates disease in the urinary tract.

Feedback control of glomerular filtration

There are two main mechanisms:

1. **Tubuloglomerular feedback**: this responds to changes in tubular fluid flow rate.
2. **Myogenic mechanism**: this responds to changes in arterial pressure.

Fig. 2.14 Composition of glomerular filtrate

Component	Glomerular filtrate
Na^+ (mmol/L)	142
K^+ (mmol/L)	4.0
Cl^- (mmol/L)	113
HCO_3^- (mmol/L)	28–30
glucose (mmol/L)	5.9
protein (g/100 mL)	0.02

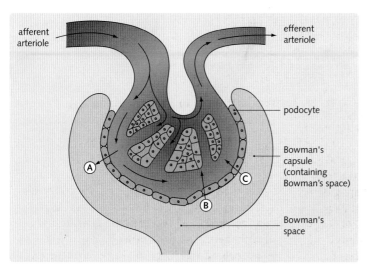

Fig. 2.13 Pressures controlling glomerular filtration into Bowman's capsule. A, Hydrostatic pressure of glomerular capillary = 50 mmHg; B, hydrostatic pressure in Bowman's space = 12 mmHg (increases fluid uptake into capillary); C, oncotic pressure of glomerular capillary = 25 mmHg (increases fluid uptake into capillary).

afferent arteriole

efferent arteriole

podocyte

Bowman's capsule (containing Bowman's space)

Bowman's space

Tubuloglomerular feedback mechanism

The GFR remains constant over a wide range of arterial pressures. Because the flow through the capillaries determines the GFR, autoregulation exists within the renal circulation. The tubuloglomerular feedback mechanism controls the GFR of each nephron by sensing the composition of the distal tubular fluid. The system has three components:

1. A luminal component that recognizes a specific variable within the tubular fluid, e.g. the macula densa cells of the tubular epithelium, which detect osmolality or the rate of Na^+ or Cl^- movement into the cells. The higher the flow of the filtrate the higher the Na^+ concentration in the cells.
2. A signal, which is sent via the juxtaglomerular cells, is triggered by a change in the NaCl concentration of distal tubular fluid.
3. An effector (angiotensin II or prostaglandins – see Chapter 3), which acts as a vasoconstrictor to contract the smooth muscle of the adjacent afferent arterioles and therefore decreases renal plasma flow, which in turn reduces GFR.

This mechanism maintains a constant GFR, thus preventing nephron overload because a high NaCl load decreases the filtration capacity of that nephron.

Myogenic mechanism

This depends on the contraction of smooth muscle cells in response to stretching. Thus, when the arterial pressure rises, the renal afferent arteriole stretches and the smooth muscle cells contract. This prevents the rise in pressure being transmitted to the glomerular capillary, so that the GFR remains unchanged.

Autoregulation of glomerular filtration relies on changes in resistance, primarily in the afferent arterioles.

TRANSPORT PROCESSES IN THE RENAL TUBULE

The ultrafiltrate produced from the glomerular filter has a similar composition to plasma and is modified by reabsorption and secretion in the tubule to produce the final urine.

Definitions

Reabsorption, secretion and excretion are defined as follows:

- **Reabsorption**: the movement of a substance from the tubular fluid back into the circulation.
- **Secretion**: the movement of substances from the blood into the tubular fluid via tubular cells (active transport) or intercellular spaces (passive process).
- **Excretion**: the removal of waste products from the blood and the net result of filtration, secretion and reabsorption of a substance.

Figure 2.15 illustrates the processes that occur in the nephron and result in excretion of a substance. Two types of solute transport are involved:

1. Paracellular movement (between cells) across the tight junctions that connect the cells. This is driven by concentration and the electrical and osmotic gradients.
2. Transcellular movement (through cells) via both the apical and basal membranes and the cell cytoplasm. Here, water follows the movement of solutes by osmosis.

Transport mechanisms

Diffusion

Diffusion is the movement of substances down their electrochemical gradient. It is a 'passive' process, as it does not require any metabolic energy or carrier molecules.

Facilitated diffusion

Like diffusion, this is also passive movement of substances along their electrochemical gradient, but it relies on a carrier molecule to transport substances across the membrane. Consequently, it is much faster than diffusion.

Primary active transport

This is an energy-dependent process in which substances cross cell membranes against their concentration and electrochemical gradients. It involves the hydrolysis of adenosine triphosphate (ATP),

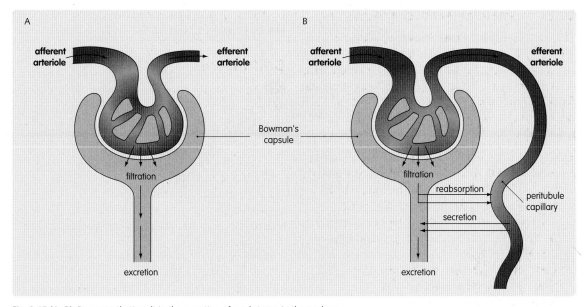

Fig. 2.15 (A, B) Processes that result in the excretion of a substance in the nephron.

which provides chemical energy for the transport mechanism.

The most important active transporter is the Na^+/K^+ ATPase pump, which is found on the basal and basolateral membranes of tubular cells. It is involved in the active transport of Na^+ from intracellular to extracellular spaces, allowing the nephron to reabsorb over 99% of the filtered Na^+. This maintains a low Na^+ concentration and a high K^+ concentration in the cell (Fig. 2.16). The other primary active transporters on the tubular cell membrane are:

- Ca^{2+} ATPase
- H^+/K^+ ATPase
- H^+ ATPase.

The ATP molecule is part of the protein structure in the primary active transporters. Energy is derived from the hydrolysis of the terminal phosphate bond of the ATP molecule to form adenosine diphosphate (ADP) and phosphate (P_i) (Fig. 2.17).

Secondary active transport

This process uses the energy produced from another process for transporting molecules (i.e. the transport of the solutes is coupled). The most important

example of this mechanism involves the Na^+/K^+ ATPase pump as the driving force for the secretion and reabsorption of other solutes in which the energy is provided by the Na^+ gradient.

The Na^+/K^+ ATPase pump creates an ionic gradient across the cell membrane, which allows the energy produced from the diffusion of Na^+ into the cell as it moves along its electrochemical gradient to be used for active transport (i.e. against their electrochemical gradients) of other solutes.

Substances can move in two directions by the following processes:

- **Symport**: energy produced by the movement of Na^+ is used to transport other substances in the same direction across the cell membrane, i.e. with the Na^+ gradient (e.g. the $Na^+/K^+/Cl^-$ co-transporter in the thick ascending limb and the Na^+/glucose in the cells of the proximal tubule cells).
- **Antiport**: movement of substances against their electrochemical gradient in the opposite direction to the Na^+ gradient (e.g. the Ca^{2+}/Na^+ and the H^+/Na^+ exchangers).

These processes are carried out by specific carrier proteins embedded in the cell membrane called transporters.

Fig. 2.16 Mechanisms of active transport in the proximal tubule cells:
• H⁺/K⁺ ATPase
• Proton pump
• Ca²⁺ ATPase
• Na⁺/K⁺ ATPase (sodium pump).

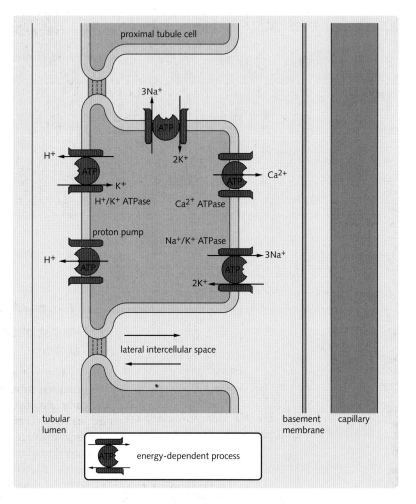

Ion channels

These are protein pores found on the epithelial cell membranes. They allow rapid transport of ions into the cell. Channels that are specific for Na^+, K^+ and Cl^- are found on the apical membrane of all the cells lining the nephron. Although transport through these channels is very fast (10^6–10^8 ions/s) there are only about 100 channels per cell, compared with the slower (100 ions/s) but more numerous active transporters (10^7 transporters per cell).

Handling of sodium by the kidney

Na^+ ions can be used to show how the filtrate is modified by various regions of the nephron to produce the excreted urine. The concentration of Na^+ in the Bowman's capsule is equal to the plasma level because Na^+ is freely filtered. Virtually all the

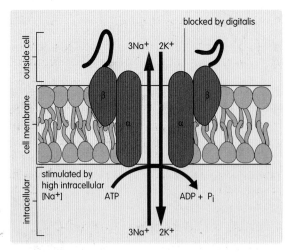

Fig. 2.17 Na⁺/K⁺ ATPase pump found in the basal membrane of the cells. It drives secondary active transport by maintaining a low Na⁺ concentration in the cells.

Fig. 2.18 Na⁺ transport along the nephron

Part of nephron	Percentage of filtered Na⁺ reabsorbed	Method of entry into the cell	Regulatory hormones
proximal tubule	65–70	Na^+ co-transport, paracellular	angiotensin II
loop of Henle	20–25	$Na^+/Cl^-/K^+$ pump (1:2:1)	aldosterone
early distal tubule	5	Na^+/Cl^- symport	aldosterone
late distal tubule and collecting ducts	5	Na^+ channels	aldosterone, atrial natriuretic peptide

Na⁺ that is filtered into the nephron is reabsorbed back into the circulation, with only 1% or less of the filtered Na⁺ being excreted in the urine. This is important not only to preserve Na⁺ levels in the body but also because the reabsorption processes of glucose, amino acids, water, lactate, Cl^-, HCO_3^- and PO_4^{3-} ions depend on the movement of Na⁺ back into the cells of the tubule. Na⁺ transport along the nephron is shown in Figure 2.18.

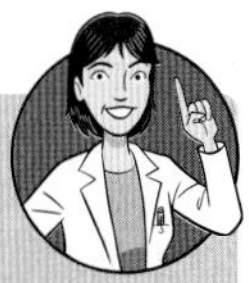

Generating Na⁺ gradients using the Na^+/K^+ATPase within the kidney is central to the reabsorption of many substances, including glucose, amino acids, water, lactate, Cl^-, HCO_3^-, and PO_4^{3-}.

THE PROXIMAL TUBULE

Microstructure

The proximal tubule is made up of two parts:

1. Pars convoluta
2. Pars recta.

The most active transport occurs in the cells of the pars convoluta. The histological structure has been discussed earlier in the chapter (see Fig. 2.6).

Transport of sodium and chloride
Movement of sodium into the lateral space

Seventy per cent of the filtered Na⁺ is reabsorbed in the proximal tubule. A lot of Na⁺ is reabsorbed in the early proximal tubule but, as the cell junctions are leaky, the concentration gradient between the filtrate and the intercellular plasma is limited. Less reabsorption occurs in the late proximal tubule, but the cell junctions are tight so a better concentration gradient is established. The primary transporter Na^+/K^+ ATPase (Na⁺ pump) on the basolateral membrane actively transports Na⁺ out of the cell into the lateral intercellular spaces between adjacent cells.

Sodium entry into the cell

This movement of Na⁺ out of the cell maintains a very low concentration of Na⁺ within the proximal tubule cells (less than 30 mmol/L). This, and the fact that there is a negative transmembrane potential relative to the lumen (−70 mV), drives Na⁺ ions to move along their concentration and electrical gradients into the cells from the tubular fluid via carrier molecules on the apical membrane. In the early proximal tubule, movement of other substances is coupled with Na⁺ transport in and out of tubule cells:

- Glucose, amino acids, PO_4^{3-} and lactate are transported by symport with Na⁺ into the cell
- H⁺ is transported by antiport out of the cell and linked to the reabsorption of HCO_3^-.

Fig. 2.19 Forces governing Na$^+$ transport in the proximal tubule

Part of proximal tubule	Electrical potential (mV)	Transport mechanism	Na$^+$ concentration (mmol/L)
tubular lumen	−2	passive (carrier molecule)	150
cell	−70	active (pump)	30
extracellular fluid	0	diffusion	150

In the late proximal tubule, Na$^+$ is mainly reabsorbed with Cl$^-$ across the cells. This occurs because the cells of the late proximal tubule have different Na$^+$ transport mechanisms and the tubular fluids have very little glucose and amino acids. The forces governing Na$^+$ transport in the proximal tubule are shown in Figure 2.19.

Chloride reabsorption

Over 60% of filtered Cl$^-$ is reabsorbed in the middle and late proximal tubule. Chloride ions enter the cells by passive reabsorption; however, the intercellular potential opposes Cl$^-$ entry into the cells in the early part of the proximal tubule. The reabsorption of glucose, amino acids and HCO$_3^-$ with Na$^+$ in the initial part of the proximal tubule creates a filtrate that becomes concentrated with Cl$^-$. The increase in Cl$^-$ produces a diffusion gradient, which allows movement of the ions into the intercellular space or directly into the cell:

- Most Cl$^-$ entry is via the tight junctions between cells along with Na$^+$
- A small amount of Cl$^-$ enters by antiport with HCO$_3^-$ and HCOO$^-$ (formate).

Water reabsorption

Seventy per cent of the filtered water is reabsorbed in the proximal tubule. This is driven by a transtubular osmotic gradient, created by solute reabsorption into the lateral intercellular spaces (Fig. 2.20). This leaves a dilute solution, which causes an increase in the hydrostatic pressure, so fluid moves by osmosis through the basement membrane into the peritubular capillary. This movement is also driven by the high oncotic pressure in the peritubular capillary because of the high plasma protein concentration created by the filtration process in the glomerulus.

The fluid leaving the proximal tubule is isosmotic because both ions and water move out of the filtrate together. The proximal tubule has no concentrating capacity.

Transport of other solutes in the proximal tubule

Glucose

Normal plasma glucose concentration is 2.5–5.5 mmol/L. Usually, 0.2–0.5 mmol of glucose is filtered every minute. An increase in the plasma glucose concentration results in a proportional increase in the amount of glucose filtered. Virtually all filtered glucose is reabsorbed in the proximal tubule, unless the amount of filtered glucose exceeds the resorptive capacity of the cells. Glucose is transported into the proximal tubule cells by symport against its concentration gradient. It is driven by the energy released from the transport of Na$^+$ down its electrochemical gradient because the Na$^+$/K$^+$ ATPase pump on the basolateral membrane maintains a low Na$^+$ concentration and negative potential within the cell (Fig. 2.21). This is an example of secondary active transport. The transport ratio is:

- 1:1 Na$^+$: glucose in the pars convoluta
- 2:1 Na$^+$: glucose in the pars recta.

T_m is the maximum tubular resorptive capacity for a solute (i.e. the point of saturation for the carriers), and this value can be calculated for glucose. All nephrons have different thresholds for glucose reabsorption (nephron heterogeneity). There is a limited number of Na$^+$/glucose carrier molecules, so glucose reabsorption is T_m limited. Figure 2.22 shows

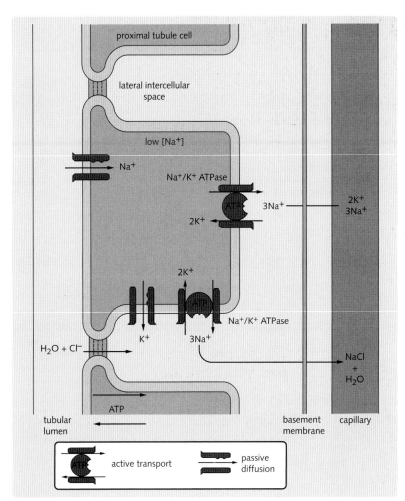

Fig. 2.20 Na$^+$ transport processes in the proximal tubule. Sodium entry into the cell is driven by its concentration gradient set up by the Na$^+$/K$^+$ ATPase pump found on the basal membrane.

that the lowest renal threshold of glucose is at a plasma glucose concentration of 10 mmol/L. At this level, filtered glucose will begin to be excreted in the urine (glycosuria). If the plasma glucose concentration increases further even those nephrons with highest resorptive capacity become saturated, and glucose is excreted. Urinary glucose increases in parallel with plasma glucose. The T_m for glucose is exceeded in all nephrons when the plasma glucose concentration is >20 mmol/L.

Glycosuria occurs if:

- The filtered load exceeds the renal threshold
- T_m for glucose is lower than normal.

Amino acids

Amino acids are the basic unit of proteins and are absorbed constantly from the gut. The plasma

If plasma glucose rises above 10 mmol/L (as in diabetes), glycosuria will develop. However, glycosuria may also occur in non-diabetic people with normal blood sugar levels as a result of certain inherited renal tubule disorders. This is called renal glycosuria. Renal glycosuria also happens in pregnancy because the T_m for glucose falls, and glucose is excreted in the urine. A glucose tolerance test may be required to differentiate renal glycosuria from diabetes.

concentration of amino acids is 2.5–3.5 mmol/L. They are small molecules that filter easily through the glomerulus, with most reabsorption occurring in the proximal tubule. The transport is a secondary active process (by symport with Na$^+$) and is driven

Fig. 2.21 Active transport of glucose in the proximal tubule (pars convoluta). This occurs against a concentration gradient.

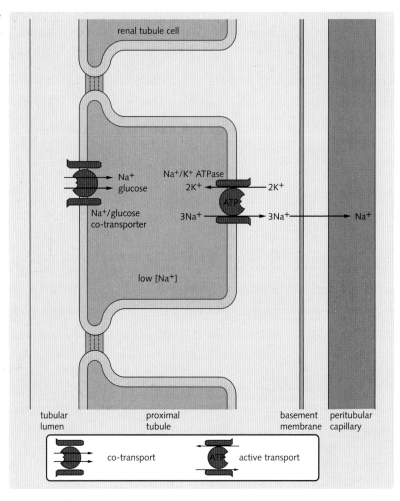

Fig. 2.22 Relation between plasma concentration, filtration, reabsorption and excretion of glucose (glomerular filtration rate = 100 mL/min). T_m is exceeded in nephrons with plasma glucose >10 mmol/L and for all nephrons when plasma glucose >20 mmol/L (nephron heterogeneity gives rise to 'splay' on the curve).

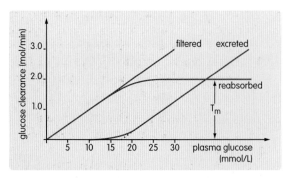

by Na^+/K^+ ATPase, as with glucose. There are at least five different transport systems coupled with Na^+ and these are responsible for the movement of different types of amino acid residue. This is a T_m-limited process, so amino aciduria results if the reabsorption mechanism is saturated or if the reabsorption mechanism is defective (e.g. in Fanconi's syndrome).

Phosphate

Phosphate (PO_4^{3-}) salts are essential for the structure of bones and teeth. Eighty per cent of the body's PO_4^{3-} content is in bone and 20% is in the intracellular fluid (ICF). It is filtered easily at the glomerulus; 80% is then reabsorbed in the proximal tubule and the remaining 20% is excreted in urine.

The kidneys play an important role in the regulation of PO_4^{3-}. The amount filtered is proportional to the plasma PO_4^{3-} concentration. Therefore, any increase in plasma PO_4^{3-} concentration (>1.2 mmol/L) leads to an increase in the amount filtered and excreted, which is how plasma PO_4^{3-} levels are controlled. A fall in GFR will result in increased plasma PO_4^{3-} concentration. Reabsorption of PO_4^{3-} occurs with Na^+ ions (two Na^+ for every PO_4^{3-} ion) at the apical membrane of the tubular cells.

PO_4^{3-} is an important urinary buffer for H^+ and its excretion is influenced by:

- Parathyroid hormone (increases excretion)
- Vitamin D (decreases excretion)
- Acidosis (increases excretion)
- Glucocorticoids (increases excretion).

Urea

Urea is the end-product of protein metabolism, which occurs in the liver. Urea is transported to the kidneys via the blood. It is a small molecule that is filtered freely at the glomerulus. The normal plasma concentration of urea is 2.5–7.5 mmol/L. Urea concentration increases in the filtrate as a result of Na^+, Cl^- and water reabsorption. This allows passive reabsorption of 40–50% of urea along its concentration gradient; 50–60% of the filtered urea is excreted in the urine. ADH increases the permeability of the inner medullary collecting ducts to urea. The distal tubule and the outer medullary ducts are impermeable to urea.

Bicarbonate

HCO_3^- is vital for the maintenance of acid–base balance within the body. The plasma concentration of HCO_3^- is 20–30 mmol/L. The kidney plays an important part in pH regulation by controlling the plasma HCO_3^- concentration. The proximal tubule reabsorbs 80% of the filtered HCO_3^- (Fig. 2.23), the remaining 20% being taken up in the distal tubule and collecting ducts. Reabsorption of HCO_3^- is coupled to Na^+ transport.

Mechanism of HCO_3^- reabsorption

Na^+ reabsorption on the apical membrane drives H^+ secretion by the tubular cells. H^+ combines with HCO_3^- ions to form H_2CO_3 (carbonic acid). Carbonic anhydrase (CA) on the brush border of the cells catalyses the dissociation of H_2CO_3 to $H_2O + CO_2$ within the tubular lumen. Both H_2O and CO_2 diffuse freely into the cell, where they re-form H_2CO_3, this process being catalysed by intracellular CA. HCO_3^- and Na^+ are actively transported out of the cell across the basolateral membrane. H^+ is secreted out of the cell into the tubular lumen and recycled to allow continuation of this cycle (see Fig. 2.25).

Sulphate

The normal plasma concentration of sulphate is 1–1.5 mmol/L. Sulphate reabsorption is T_m limited and this is an important mechanism in regulating its plasma concentration.

Potassium

The plasma concentration of potassium is 4–5 mmol/L. Approximately 70% of K^+ is reabsorbed in the proximal tubule, mostly by passive paracellular reabsorption across the tight junctions between tubular cells. K^+ can be secreted or reabsorbed in the nephron. Excretion of the filtered K^+ can vary from 1% to 110% depending on:

- Dietary intake of potassium
- Acid–base status
- Aldosterone levels.

K^+ reabsorption occurs mainly in the thick ascending loop of Henle by co-transport of $Na^+/K^+/Cl^-$ on the luminal membrane. Reabsorption of K^+ occurs in the distal tubule during severe dietary depletion of K^+.

Secretion by the proximal tubule

Secretion is the movement of solutes from the proximal tubule cells into the tubular fluid. It can be active (i.e. require energy) or passive. These processes are T_m limited or gradient time-limited.

There are three T_m-limited secretory mechanisms for:

1. Strong organic bases (e.g. choline, histamine and thiamine), which are secreted in the pars convoluta.
2. Strong organic acids (e.g. penicillin, p-aminohippuric acid (PAH)), which are secreted in the pars recta as the substances move out from the peritubular capillaries.
3. Ethylenediamine tetra-acetic acid (EDTA).

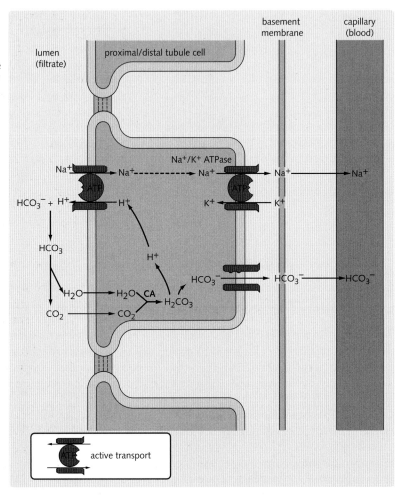

Fig. 2.23 HCO_3^- reabsorption in the proximal tubule cells. Secreted H^+ combines with HCO_3^- to form carbonic acid. This is broken down by carbonic anhydrase (CA) in the brush border to CO_2 and H_2O, which diffuse freely into the cell. The process is reversed inside the cell to re-form HCO_3^-.

The substances handled by gradient time-limited mechanisms include:

- H^+: secretion of H^+ depends on the transport of Na^+ and the reabsorption of HCO_3^-. The movement of H^+ out of the cells occurs by an antiport with Na^+ on the apical membrane using a specific transporter.
- K^+: this varies, and depends on diet, aldosterone levels, acid–base status and the urine flow.

THE LOOP OF HENLE

Role of the loop of Henle

The loop of Henle reabsorbs 20% of the filtered Na^+ and 15% of tubular water. As filtrate flows through the loop of Henle, reabsorption of NaCl in the thick ascending limb produces a hypertonic interstitial fluid in the surrounding medulla. This creates a concentration gradient and water moves passively out of the thin descending limb.

The tubular fluid is isotonic to the plasma on entering the loop of Henle; however, by the time it leaves the loop it is hypotonic because ion reabsorption occurs within the loop. This mechanism allows urine to be concentrated, using the least amount of energy, because water is then reabsorbed passively from the collecting ducts into the hypertonic interstitium of the medulla.

Structure of the loop of Henle

The different components of the loop are functionally separate units, each with its own specific properties.

Thin descending limb

The thin descending limb is lined by thin, flat cells that have minimal cytoplasmic specialization. It is permeable to water, Na^+ and Cl^-. Water is reabsorbed passively down a concentration gradient caused by the hypertonic interstitium of the medulla. NaCl moves into the lumen and water moves out of the lumen into the interstitium, allowing the tubular fluid to come into equilibrium with the interstitium.

- The juxtamedullary nephrons have long, thin limbs that extend deep into the inner medulla.
- The cortical nephrons only just enter the medulla and some are situated entirely in the cortex.

Thin ascending limb

The thin ascending limb has a similar structure to the thin descending limb but is impermeable to water and has minimal NaCl transport occurring within the cells.

Thick ascending limb

The thick ascending limb consists of large cells with mitochondria, which generate energy for the active transport of Na^+ (20% of filtered Na^+ is reabsorbed in the loop of Henle) and Cl^- ions from the tubular fluid into the interstitium. As a result, the filtrate becomes progressively diluted (this part of the tubule is impermeable to water). There is co-transport (symport) of Na^+, Cl^- and K^+ (in the ratio 1:2:1 – so the pump is electrochemically neutral) on the apical membrane. This transport process is driven by the Na^+ gradient across the cell membrane. Na^+ is removed from the cell by the Na^+/K^+ ATPase pump on the basolateral membrane and K^+ and Cl^- diffuse passively out as a result of Na^+ movement; however, most of the K^+ leaks back into the cell and tubular lumen. Overall, NaCl accumulates in the medullary interstitium. Figure 2.24 shows the transport processes in the loop of Henle; the inset shows the transport of ions in the cells in the thick ascending limb of the loop of Henle.

Countercurrent multiplication

Any mechanism that will concentrate urine must be able to reabsorb water from the tubular fluid as it passes through the collecting ducts. The loop of Henle, which acts as a countercurrent multiplier, produces a hypertonic medulla by pooling NaCl in the interstitium, which favours the subsequent movement of water out of the collecting ducts (under the regulation of ADH). Each portion of the loop contributes to the effectiveness of this system.

The mechanism of the countercurrent multiplier is illustrated in Figure 2.25. The thick, ascending limb can maintain a difference of $200\,mOsmol/kgH_2O$ between the tubular fluid and the interstitium at any point along its length. The maximum osmolality of the interstitium is $1400\,mOsmol/kg\,H_2O$ (normal plasma osmolality is $300\,mOsmol/kg\,H_2O$) at the tip of the loop. The fluid leaving the loop of Henle is hypotonic ($100\,mOsmol/kg\,H_2O$).

Role of urea and vasa recta

The countercurrent mechanism requires an environment in which the waste products and water are cleared without disturbing the solutes that maintain the medullary hypertonicity. This exchange is provided by the vasa recta capillary system derived from the efferent arterioles of the longer juxtaglomerular nephrons. It does not require metabolic energy.

The capillaries have a hairpin arrangement surrounding the loop of Henle and are permeable to water and solutes. As the descending vessels pass through the medulla they absorb solutes such as Na^+, urea and Cl^-. Water moves along its osmotic gradient out of the capillaries. At the tip of the loop the capillary blood has the same osmolality as the interstitium, and an osmotic equilibrium is reached. The capillaries that ascend with the corresponding loop of Henle contain very viscous concentrated blood as a result of the earlier loss of water from the capillaries. A consequent increase in oncotic pressure because of the concentration of plasma proteins favours the movement of water back into the blood vessel from the interstitium. However, most of the NaCl is retained in the interstitium to maintain the hypertonic medullary environment.

The collecting tubules pass through the cortex and medulla. They consist of two functionally different parts:

1. The cortical collecting ducts
2. The medullary (inner and outer) collecting ducts.

Both parts are impermeable to NaCl. The permeability to water and urea (only in the inner medullary

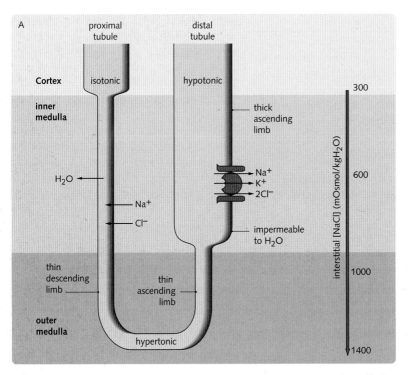

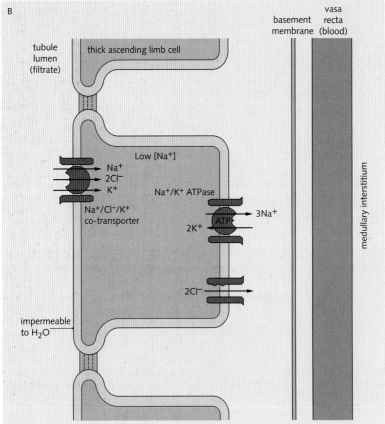

Fig. 2.24 (A) Transport processes in the loop of Henle. (B) Transport of ions in the thick ascending limb.

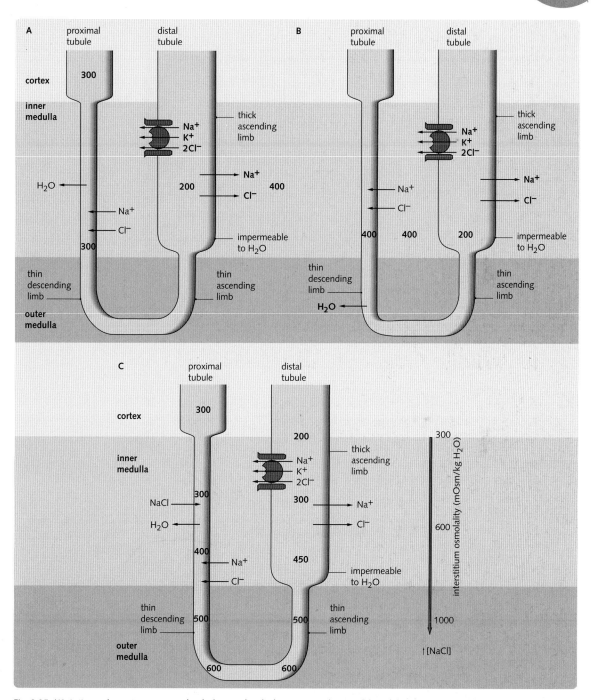

Fig. 2.25 (A) Active reabsorption occurs in the thick ascending limb, increasing the osmolality of the medulla (400 mOsmol/kg H$_2$O). The tubular fluid therefore decreases in osmolality (200 mOsmol/kg H$_2$O). (B) The increase in interstitial osmolality stimulates H$_2$O to leave the descending limb into the medulla. At the same time, increased interstitial osmolality results in passive diffusion of NaCl out of the medulla into the tubule until equilibrium is reached (400 mOsmol/kg H$_2$O). (C) The fluid in the tubule is progressively concentrated in descending the tubule as it comes into equilibrium with its surroundings (maximum value of 600 mOsmol/kg H$_2$O at the tip of the loop) and hence progressively diluted as it ascends the loop. This is all due to active NaCl reabsorption in the thick ascending limb (and some passive movement of NaCl in the ascending limb). Therefore a longitudinal gradient is set up, with greatest osmolality in the lower medulla and least in the cortex.

Fig. 2.26 Countercurrent exchanger as it passes through the medulla. The descending vessels of the vasa recta lose water as they pass through the hypertonic medulla. As a result of increasing oncotic pressure in the ascending vessels, water is reabsorbed passively back into the blood vessels from the interstitium as water uptake occurs in the collecting ducts under the influence of antidiuretic hormone (ADH). Because of this uptake of water by the vasa recta, the high osmolality of the medullary interstitium is maintained and this hypertonic environment allows continued concentration of the tubular fluid in the collecting duct.

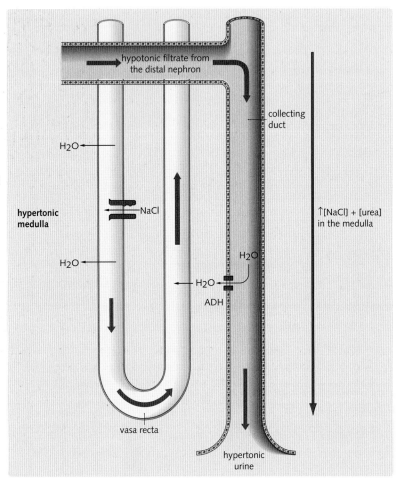

collecting ducts) varies according to the presence of ADH. ADH increases the permeability to water and thus controls the concentration of the urine produced. ADH acts to increase water uptake in the cortical collecting tubules resulting in the production of a more concentrated urine.

The water reabsorbed in the medullary part of the collecting ducts is taken up by the vasa recta to prevent dilution of the medullary interstitium, which is crucial to the function of the distal nephron and the concentration of urine.

Although about 20% of the initial glomerular filtrate enters the distal nephron, only 5% enters the medullary collecting ducts. This is mainly due to water reabsorption in the cortical tubules.

The structure, location and function of the loop of Henle has a central role in the development of a hypertonic gradient in the medulla. This allows urine to be concentrated as it passes through the collecting tubules.

Figure 2.26 shows the countercurrent exchanger and the collecting duct as it passes through the medulla.

Although urea is impermeable in the cortical collecting tubules, ADH affects the permeability of urea within the medullary cortical tubules. Urea,

along with NaCl, helps maintain medullary hypertonicity as follows:

- 50% of the filtered urea is reabsorbed in the
  proximal tubule with Na^+.
- The tubular concentration of urea increases as it
  diffuses out of the medullary interstitium into
  the lumen down its concentration gradient.
- The remaining urea becomes further
  concentrated within the tubular lumen as water
  and other solutes are reabsorbed into the cells
  of the distal tubule and the cortical collecting
  tubules, a process aided by the fact that
  these parts of the nephron are impermeable
  to urea.
- The concentration of urea in the medullary
  collecting tubules is so high that it diffuses out
  of the lumen into the interstitium, thus
  increasing the concentration of urea in the
  medulla and recycling it. This occurs in the
  presence of ADH.

A high-protein diet increases the amount of urea in
the blood for excretion as a result of increased
metabolism. Consequently, there is more urea in the
medullary interstitium, resulting in a higher urine
osmolality.

ADH is released from the posterior pituitary in
response to increases in ECF osmolality. Diabetes
insipidus results from the failure of action or secretion
of ADH, and an inability to reabsorb water. Syndrome
of inappropriate ADH secretion (SIADH) results from
an abnormally high amount of ADH release and an
inappropriately concentrated urine. (These are dealt
with in more detail in Chapter 3.)

Regulation of urine concentration

ADH levels within the body determine the concentration and volume of urine:

- Average daily urine volume is 1.0–1.5 L (normal
  range 400 mL to 2–3 L)
- Average urine osmolality is 450 mOsmol/kg H_2O
  (normal range 60–1400 mOsmol/kg H_2O).

The presence of cortisol is vital for the action of
ADH. Aldosterone is also very important in concentrating urine because it affects Na^+ reabsorption. By
increasing Na^+ uptake in the cortical collecting
tubules more water is passively reabsorbed, so urine
volume decreases and osmolality increases (ADH is
considered further in Chapter 3).

Objectives

By the end of the chapter you should be able to:

- Define clearance. Explain how it is measured and what its units are
- Explain the relevance of clearance ratios
- Describe how to measure the glomerular filtration rate and renal blood flow. Discuss how this varies with age
- Outline the factors that affect creatinine clearance
- Define autoregulation and explain how it is achieved
- Explain what osmoreceptors are, where they are located and what their function is
- Briefly describe the synthesis, storage and function of antidiuretic hormone (ADH)
- Describe how the kidneys' ability to concentrate or dilute urine is altered in disease
- Summarize the importance of the renin–angiotensin–aldosterone system
- Outline the mechanisms controlling Na^+ reabsorption
- Describe the effective circulating volume and explain how this is regulated
- List the causes and the clinical presentation of syndrome of inappropriate ADH secretion (SIADH)
- Distinguish the two types of diabetes insipidus and explain how they differ
- State the normal pH range. Outline how and why it is tightly controlled
- Explain what a 'buffer' is, and name the main buffering system in the body and describe how it works
- Explain how metabolic acidosis and metabolic alkalosis are differentiated by arterial blood gas results and give an outline of how you would correct each of them
- Discuss the significance of the anion gap
- Describe the distribution of K^+ within the body compartments and explain why it is important to keep this distribution constant
- Explain the relation between plasma calcium and phosphate. Describe the influence of three factors involved in their regulation
- Discuss when erythropoietin release is stimulated and what its effects are.

RENAL BLOOD FLOW AND THE GLOMERULAR FILTRATION RATE

Measurement of glomerular filtration rate

Clearance

Clearance (C) is the volume of plasma that is cleared of a substance in a unit time. It is a measure of the kidney's ability to remove a substance from the plasma and excrete it. The clearance of a substance x is:

$$\text{Clearance of } \chi \text{ (mL/min)} C_x = \frac{\substack{\text{urine concentration} \\ \text{of } \chi \text{ (mg/mL)} \\ U_x \times \text{urine flow rate} \\ \text{(mL/min) } V}}{\substack{\text{plasma} \\ \text{concentration of} \\ \chi \text{ (mg/mL) } P_x}}$$

Clearance of a substance will provide an accurate estimate of the glomerular filtration rate (GFR) if that substance 'follows' the filtrate without being altered by the kidney (i.e. is not reabsorbed, secreted, synthesized or metabolized by the kidney). Inulin is such a substance:

- It is a polysaccharide of molecular weight 5500
- It is not normally found within the body, so is introduced into the body by injection or intravenous infusion
- It passes into the glomerular filtrate but is not reabsorbed, secreted, synthesized or metabolized by the kidney – so all inulin filtered by the glomerulus is excreted in the urine. Inulin clearance can be used to assess glomerular function in disease.

Normal inulin clearance is equal to the GFR, i.e. $120 \text{ mL/min}/1.73 \text{ m}^2$ body surface area (this varies with body size). However, measurement of inulin clearance is complicated and is rarely used to assess GFR in routine clinical practice. Instead, creatinine clearance is used as an estimate of GFR. Creatinine is found in the body; it is produced during muscle metabolism:

Phosphocreatine + ADP $\xrightarrow{\text{creatine phosphokinase}}$ creatine + ATP

Creatine + H_2O $\longrightarrow$ creatinine

Plasma creatinine levels remain constant if renal function, muscle mass and metabolism are stable. Plasma creatinine is commonly used to indicate renal function. Its exact value depends not only on renal function but also upon muscle mass and therefore age, sex and size. It has a reciprocal relationship with GFR (see Fig. 3.1).

Like inulin, creatinine is filtered freely and is not affected or produced by the kidney. It can therefore be used to measure GFR.

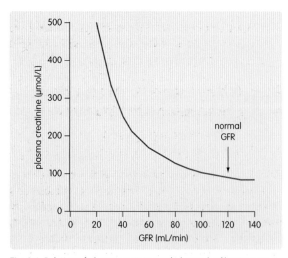

Fig. 3.1 Relation of plasma creatinine and glomerular filtration rate (GFR). Normal GFR is typically 90–120 mL/min (from Koeppen BM, Stanton B 1996 Renal physiology, 2nd edn. Mosby Year Book).

Estimated glomerular filtration rate (eGFR)

Plasma creatinine levels do not accurately reflect renal function. GFR is widely accepted as the best measure of kidney function; however, it is difficult to measure and in clinical practice it is infrequently utilized. Instead the GFR may be estimated using a simple formula (the most commonly used of which is the MDRD equation). MDRD eGFR is calculated from the age, sex, race and creatinine level of the patient and is now commonly used to classify chronic kidney disease (see Chapter 6).

Clearance ratios

Information about how the kidney clears a particular substance, x (C_x), can be obtained by comparing its clearance with that of inulin (C_{in}):

- Substances with clearance values greater than inulin clearance ($C_x > C_{in}$): the substance enters the renal tubule by glomerular filtration and tubular secretion (e.g. *p*-aminohippuric acid (PAH)).
- Substances with clearance values lower than inulin clearance ($C_x < C_{in}$): the substance is either not freely filtered at the glomerulus, or is freely filtered but then reabsorbed from the tubule.

Measurement of renal blood flow

The Fick principle states that the amount of substance x removed from plasma by the kidney in 1 min is equal to the amount appearing in urine in 1 min. This is illustrated by the formula:

(Arterial concentration of χ A_x – venous concentration of χ V_x) × renal plasma flow (RPF)

RPF = urinary flow rate V × Urinary concentration of χ U_x

PAH is an organic acid that is filtered at the glomerulus and secreted by the proximal tubules (transport maximum (T_m) limited). Thus, the amount of PAH excreted equals the amount filtered and secreted in the kidney. If the T_m for PAH is not exceeded, at least 90% is removed from the blood as it passes through the kidney in a normal individual. Therefore the clearance of PAH can be used to measure RPF (Fig. 3.2). If plasma PAH concentration is less than 0.1 mg/mL, T_m for PAH is not exceeded. The extraction of PAH from the blood approaches

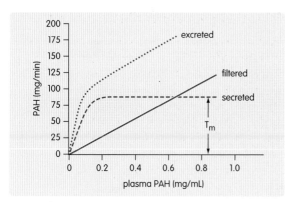

Fig. 3.2 Filtration, secretion and excretion of *p*-aminohippuric acid (PAH) compared with its plasma concentration.

- When [PAH] is greater than T_m
- In chronic renal failure
- In tubular dysfunction.

PAH clearance provides a non-invasive estimate of the renal plasma flow.

Other methods of measuring RBF (not used routinely in clinical practice) include the inert gas 'washout' technique and the isotope uptake technique.

Filtration fraction

This is the percentage of plasma flow passing the glomerulus that is filtered:

$$\text{Filtration fraction} = \frac{\text{GFR}}{\text{RPF}}$$

In a normal man:

$$\text{Filtration fraction} = \frac{120}{600} = 20\%$$

Fractional excretion (FE)

This is a measure of net reabsorption or net secretion of a substance (x):

$$FE_x = \frac{\text{mass excreted}}{\text{mass filtered}}$$

$$= \frac{(U_x \times V)}{(\text{GFR} \times P_x)}$$

FE is often expressed as a percentage. Therefore, if the FE is 0.24, 24% of the filtered mass is excreted and 76% undergoes net reabsorption.

Regulation of renal blood flow and glomerular filtration rate

- RBF is 1100 mL/min (RPF is 600 mL/min)
- GFR is 120 mL/min.

100%, so venous concentration of PAH is zero (V_{PAH}) and C_{PAH} equals RPF.

When the excretion of PAH is 100%, if P_{PAH} = the plasma concentration of PAH, U_{PAH} = the urine concentration of PAH and V = urinary flow rate:

$$\text{RPF} \times P_{PAH} = V \times U_{PAH}$$

or

$$\text{RPF} = \frac{V \times U_{PAH}}{P_{PAH}} = C_{PAH}$$

The normal RPF is 600 mL/min.

Renal blood flow (RBF) can be obtained from RPF by using the haematocrit (the percentage of total blood volume that is made of erythrocytes). The haematocrit is 45%, so 55% of blood is made up of plasma:

$$\text{RBF} = \text{RPF} \times \frac{100}{55}$$

$$= 600 \times \frac{100}{55}$$

$$= 1100 \text{ mL/min}$$

However, C_{PAH} is not an exact measurement of RPF. This is because renal blood flows to the capsule, perirenal fat and medulla, as well as to the glomeruli and tubules. Therefore, PAH clearance estimates cortical plasma flow and is usually referred to as effective RPF (ERPF).

If PAH excretion is reduced significantly, C_{PAH} becomes a less reliable marker of RPF unless this is taken into account. Excretion is reduced:

Both remain fairly constant because of autoregulation, which involves changes in tone of the afferent and efferent arterioles (Fig. 3.3). Over the autoregulatory range of perfusion pressures (90–200 mmHg), blood flow is independent of perfusion pressure so, as the perfusion pressure increases, resistance to flow increases (Fig. 3.4). Two mechanisms are involved in autoregulation:

Fig. 3.3 The regulation of renal blood flow (RBF) and glomerular filtration rate (GFR) by vasoconstriction of arterioles.

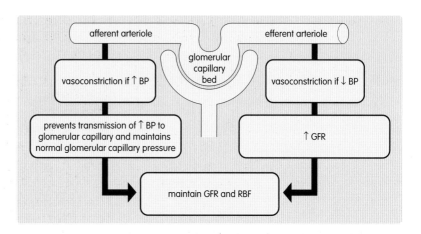

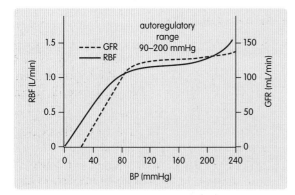

Fig. 3.4 Autoregulation of glomerular filtration rate (GFR) and renal blood flow (RBF).

1. Myogenic mechanism
2. Tubuloglomerular feedback mechanism.

Myogenic mechanism

An increase in pressure (caused by an increase in blood flow) stimulates stretch receptors in smooth muscle fibres in the vessel wall. This causes reflex contraction of smooth muscle fibres, resulting in vessel vasoconstriction. There is an increased resistance to flow so, overall, RBF remains constant.

Tubuloglomerular feedback mechanism

By monitoring the NaCl concentration at the macula densa pressure/flow changes within the kidney can be detected. Changes in the pressure/flow are transmitted from the macula densa to cells in the juxtaglomerular apparatus (JGA), which produce vasoactive substances to counteract the changes and thereby regulates GFR within a certain range. For example, if GFR rises, the tubular flow rate also increases, so less Na^+ and Cl^- are reabsorbed and a higher concentration is detected at the macula densa. This stimulates the JGA to release vasoconstrictor substances which reduce GFR. The main mediator involved in this mechanism is angiotensin II and, to a lesser extent, prostaglandins and adenosine.

Renal blood flow and systemic blood pressure

Autoregulation maintains a constant blood flow to the kidneys despite changes in blood pressure. However, the blood flow itself is not always constant; for example, acute haemorrhage results in increased sympathetic activity to the kidney (and other parts of the body). This leads to vasoconstriction and consequently decreased blood flow. Intrarenal vasodilator prostaglandins are produced to prevent excessive vasoconstriction and renal perfusion is thus maintained.

Regulation of GFR involves other vasoactive substances, which are found in the walls of blood vessels. These are summarized in Figure 3.5.

Age-related changes in renal blood flow and glomerular filtration rate

Age-related changes in RBF and GFR (Fig. 3.6) are as follows:

- Week 10 of gestation (in utero): filtration of fluid and urine production begin; this contributes to the amniotic fluid.

- Newborn: GFR ~25 mL/min/1.73 m² body surface area. RBF ~5% of cardiac output – this increases progressively during the first year.
- 1 month old: progressive increase in GFR (PAH cannot be used to measure RBF because tubular secretion is not developed, so extraction of PAH is less than 100%).
- By 1 year of age: GFR reaches adult values (120 mL/min).
- Adults: RBF ~20% of cardiac output.
- Old age: GFR decreases progressively from about 40 years of age.

BODY FLUID OSMOLALITY

Concepts of osmolality

Body weight remains relatively constant from day to day because total body water remains constant. The normal intake and output of water are discussed in Chapter 1. At least 400 mL/day of urine must be produced for the kidney to maintain homeostasis.

The normal plasma osmolality (P_{osm}) is 285–295 mOsmol/kg H_2O. This is strictly regulated

Fig. 3.5 Vasoactive substances found in the blood vessel walls	
Vasodilator	**Vasoconstrictor**
prostaglandins (PGs)	adenosine
nitric oxide (NO)	angiotensin II
dopamine (DA)	antidiuretic hormone (ADH)
bradykinin	endothelin
	norepinephrine (NE)

and an increase or decrease of 3 mOsmol/kg H_2O will stimulate the body's osmolality regulation mechanism.

> In children younger than 5 years, bed wetting may be normal. However, repeated bedwetting in children over the age of 5 years may indicate a pathological cause and is called nocturnal enuresis. It occurs in about 10% of children aged 10, affecting boys more than girls. One cause is a reduction in circulating nocturnal antidiuretic hormone (ADH) levels. This may be managed by many methods, including the use of an ADH analogue called desmopressin, administered by a nasal spray.

Osmoreceptors

Osmoreceptors detect changes in the plasma osmolality and are located in the supraoptic and paraventricular areas of the anterior hypothalamus. Their blood supply is the internal carotid artery. They have two functions:

1. To regulate the release of antidiuretic hormone (ADH, also known as vasopressin)
2. To regulate thirst (this also depends on other osmoreceptors in the lateral preoptic area of the hypothalamus).

Figure 3.7 illustrates the role of ADH in maintaining osmolality.

Sensitivity of osmoreceptors to osmotic changes caused by different solutes

Na⁺ and other associated anions are the main constituents that determine plasma osmolality. Water loss alters the Na⁺ concentration. Other solutes without the addition or loss of water can

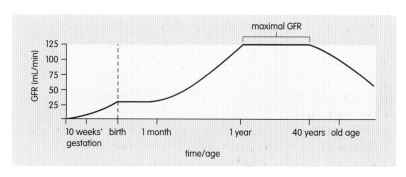

Fig. 3.6 Age-related changes in glomerular filtration rate (GFR).

Fig. 3.7 Role of antidiuretic hormone (ADH) in maintaining osmolality. The lateral preoptic area of the hypothalamus regulates thirst. The supraoptic and paraventricular nuclei are involved in ADH release from the posterior pituitary. ECF, extracellular fluid.

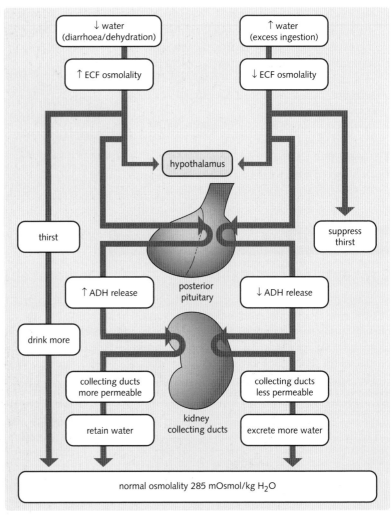

also change the osmolality. Not all solutes stimulate the osmoreceptors to the same degree – this depends on how easily they can cross the cell membrane (i.e. their ability to cause cellular dehydration).

Antidiuretic hormone (vasopressin)

Synthesis and storage

ADH is a peptide hormone synthesized in the supra-optic nucleus of the hypothalamus as a large precursor molecule. It is transported to the posterior pituitary gland, where its synthesis is completed and it is stored until release (Fig. 3.8).

Release

A rise in plasma osmolality triggers ADH release. Action potentials in the neurons from the hypothalamus (which contains ADH) depolarize the axon membrane, resulting in Ca^{2+} influx, fusion of secretory granules with the axon membrane and the release of ADH and neurophysin into the bloodstream.

Cellular actions

ADH has two functions:

1. To reduce water excretion (V_2 receptor mediated)
2. To stimulate blood vessel vasoconstriction (V_1 receptor mediated).

44

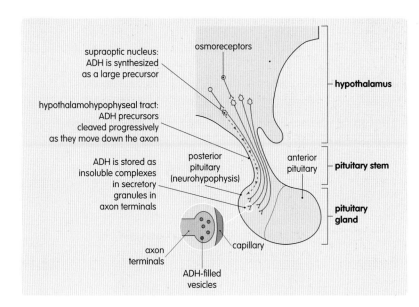

Fig. 3.8 Synthesis and storage of antidiuretic hormone (ADH). CNS, central nervous system.

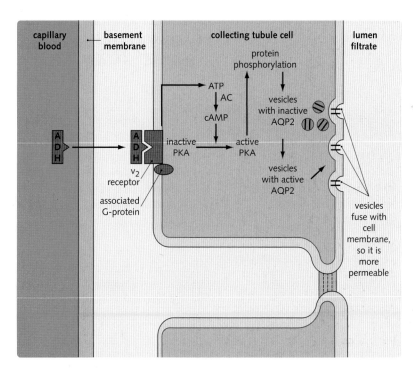

Fig. 3.9 Actions of antidiuretic hormone (ADH) in the collecting tubule. AC, adenylate cyclase; cAMP, cyclic adenosine monophosphate; PKA, protein kinase; AQP2, aquaporin 2 water channel.

Aquaporins

When present on the peritubular side of the collecting tubule cell (Fig. 3.9), ADH causes intracellular water channels (aquaporins) to fuse with the luminal membrane. There are at present 11 known members of the mammalian aquaporin gene family which encode for proteins involved in the transport of water or small molecules. In the kidney, aquaporin 2 (AQP2) resides in intracellular vesicles and is trafficked to the luminal membrane on stimulation. ADH triggers this by binding to V_2 receptors on the basal membrane. These are G-protein-coupled

45

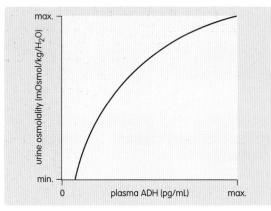

Fig. 3.10 Urine osmolality in relation to plasma antidiuretic hormone (ADH) concentration (from Berne RM, Levy MN 1996 Physiology, 3rd edn. Mosby Year Book).

Fig. 3.11 Causes of syndrome of inappropriate antidiuretic hormone secretion (SIADH)

Disorder	Example of finding
CNS disorders	abscess, stroke, vasculitis (systemic lupus erythematosus)
malignancy	small cell carcinoma in lungs, duodenum, pancreas, prostate, ureter, adrenals
lung diseases	tuberculosis, pneumonia, abscess, aspergillosis
drugs	opiates, chlorpropamide, psychotropics, cytotoxics, narcotics, oxytocin
metabolic diseases	porphyria, hypothyroidism
miscellaneous	pain (postoperative), Guillain–Barré syndrome, trauma

receptors, which on activation cause fusion of the inactive vesicles with the luminal membrane. The relation between urine osmolality (mOsmol/kg) and plasma ADH concentration is shown in Figure 3.10.

ADH secretion is controlled by:

- Osmoreceptors (which detect changes in the body fluid osmolarity)
- Baroreceptors (which detect changes in blood volume, i.e. blood vessel wall 'stretch').

The osmoreceptor system is more sensitive than the baroreceptor system.

Fate of ADH

ADH must be removed rapidly from the blood once plasma osmolarity has been corrected. This is done by the liver and kidneys (50%), with less than 10% appearing in the urine; the rest is metabolized. Its short plasma half-life (10–15 min) also ensures that the duration of its effect in the blood is limited.

Drugs affecting ADH release

Drugs can:

- Increase ADH release (e.g. nicotine, ether, morphine, barbiturates)
- Inhibit ADH release (e.g. alcohol).

Syndrome of inappropriate ADH secretion (SIADH)

Occasionally ADH is secreted inappropriately by the pituitary or other areas in the body. Causes are given in Fig. 3.11. Signs and symptoms are:

- Hyponatraemia (<125 mmol/L) and low plasma osmolality (<260 mmol/L)
- Inappropriate urine osmolality: the urine concentration is higher than normal (i.e. not maximally diluted)
- Inappropriate Na^+ excretion: urinary $[Na^+]$ is greater than 20 mmol/L despite a decrease in plasma Na^+ concentration because the plasma volume is maintained by water retention (unless volume contracted or sodium restricted, which can decrease urinary Na^+).

The diagnosis should be considered in hyponatraemic patients in the absence of hypovolaemia, oedema, endocrine dysfunction, renal failure and drugs, all of which can impair water excretion.

Diabetes insipidus

This is the inability to reabsorb water from the distal part of the nephron, due to the failure of secretion or action of ADH. Symptoms are:

- Polyuria
- Polydipsia
- Low urine osmolality, i.e. dilute urine.

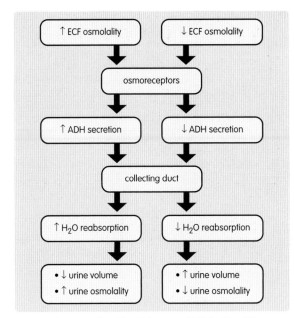

Fig. 3.12 Summary of antidiuretic hormone (ADH) action. ECF, extracellular fluid.

The causes of diabetes insipidus are:
- Neurogenic/central: impaired ADH synthesis or secretion by the hypothalamus, which might be congenital, caused by hypothalamic damage or due to pituitary tumours. It can be treated by administering ADH.
- Nephrogenic: failure of the kidneys to respond to circulating ADH, which could be caused by mutations in the gene coding for V_2 receptors, chronic pyelonephritis, polycystic kidneys or drugs such as lithium. Plasma ADH levels are normal. There is no current treatment to correct the deficit.

Diabetes insipidus can be mistaken for psychogenic polydipsia, in which large volumes of dilute urine are produced secondary to compulsive water drinking. This causes a decrease in the urine-concentrating ability because of loss of medullary tonicity.

Figure 3.12 summarizes the action of ADH.

Water clearance and reabsorption

Dehydration leads to a rise in plasma osmolality. Thus, the kidneys reabsorb 'solute-free' water from the tubules. This produces a more dilute plasma and a concentrated urine.

Excessive water intake lowers plasma osmolality. Thus, the kidneys excrete 'solute-free' water from the tubules, producing dilute urine. Dilute urine has a lower osmolality than plasma, concentrated urine has a higher osmolality than plasma, isotonic urine has the same osmolality as plasma. The osmotic clearance (C_{osm}) (Fig. 3.13) is the rate at which osmotically active substances are cleared from the plasma. If urine is isotonic, C_{osm} = urine flow (Fig. 3.13).

Effect of solute output on urine volume

The concentrating ability of the kidneys is limited, with a maximum urinary osmolality of 1400 mOsmol/kg. Thus, the amount of urine excreted per day depends on the:

- Amount of ADH
- Amount of solute excreted.

At maximum ADH concentration, large amounts of solutes can still cause a diuresis (see Fig. 3.14).

Mannitol is an osmotic diuretic that cannot be reabsorbed. It alters the kidney's concentrating ability and produces isotonic urine. In diabetes mellitus, the excess blood glucose causes an osmotic diuresis.

Adrenal steroids and urinary dilution

Adrenal insufficiency leads to impaired water excretion (i.e. mineralocorticoid and/or glucocorticoid deficiency):

- Glucocorticoid deficiency can enhance water permeability of the collecting duct
- Glucocorticoid and mineralocorticoid deficiencies increase ADH levels, resulting in an inability to produce dilute urine. This is corrected by administering adrenal steroids.

BODY FLUID VOLUME

Basic concepts
Effective circulating volume

The volume of fluid that perfuses tissues is the effective circulating volume; this needs to be kept constant. Na^+ is the major extracellular ion and affects the extracellular fluid (ECF) volume, for example, a

Fig. 3.13 Osmotic clearance. ADH, antidiuretic hormone.

$$C_{osm} = \frac{U_{osm} \times V}{P_{osm}}$$

If urine is isotonic then $\dfrac{U_{osm}}{P_{osm}} = 1$ $\therefore C_{osm} = V$

Key		
U_{osm}	=	urine osmolality
P_{osm}	=	plasma osmolality
V	=	volume
C_{osm}	=	osmotic clearance
C_{H_2O}	=	free water clearance
$T_{C_{H_2O}}$	=	free water reabsorption

If urine osmolality < plasma osmolality, i.e. dilute urine production:

$$\frac{U_{osm}}{P_{osm}} < 1 \quad \therefore C_{osm} < V$$

The urine volume has additional free water and isotonic fluid

$$\therefore V = C_{osm} + C_{H_2O}$$

Maximum C_{H_2O} = 12–15 mL/min (15–22 L/day)

If urine osmolality > plasma osmolality, i.e. concentrated urine produced:

$$\frac{U_{osm}}{P_{osm}} > 1 \quad \therefore C_{osm} > V$$

Here however, water is being excreted so

$$\therefore V = C_{osm} - T_{C_{H_2O}}$$

Water is reabsorbed here so we can substitute (C_{H_2O}) for $T_{C_{H_2O}}$

C_{H_2O} and $T_{C_{H_2O}}$ are quantitative ways of determining the ability of the kidney to excrete or conserve water

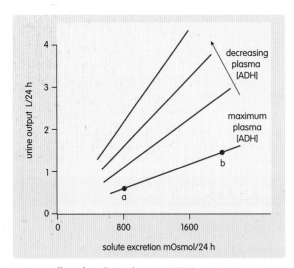

Fig. 3.14 Effect of antidiuretic hormone (ADH) on urine output. a, minimum possible urine output with a solute excretion of 800mOsmol/24h; b, minimum urine output if 2000mOsmol/24h must be excreted.

rise in ECF Na⁺ results in increased osmolality, which leads to water retention and thirst (increased drinking of water). This increases ECF volume and normalizes osmolality. Thus, the ECF volume can be regulated by controlling the body's Na⁺.

If ECF volume decreases sufficiently, intrarenal mechanisms can decrease GFR to prevent further volume loss (tubuloglomerular feedback).

Renin and angiotensin

Renin–angiotensin–aldosterone (RAA) system

The RAA system (Fig. 3.15) maintains Na⁺ balance.

Renin

Renin is an enzyme that is synthesized and stored in the JGA in the kidneys. A fall in plasma Na⁺ leads to a fall in ECF volume, causing the release of renin by:

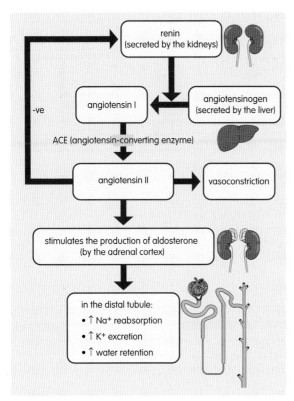

Fig. 3.15 The renin–angiotensin–aldosterone system. –ve, negative feedback.

Conversion of angiotensinogen to angiotensin

Renin acts on angiotensinogen (α_2-globulin), which splits off angiotensin I (a decapeptide). Angiotensin-converting enzyme (ACE) in the lungs then removes two amino acids to produce angiotensin II (an octapeptide). Angiotensin II:

- Stimulates the zona glomerulosa of the adrenal cortex to release aldosterone
- Directly vasoconstricts arterioles within the kidney (efferent > afferent)
- Directly increases Na^+ reabsorption from the proximal tubule
- Releases ADH
- Stimulates thirst
- Provides negative feedback to the JGA cells, and therefore affects renin release (Fig. 3.15).

In addition to the generation of circulating angiotensin II, the local generation of angiotensin II by ACE (within the tissues) might have an important pathogenic role. ACE inhibitors are used to treat high blood pressure. They decrease the production of angiotensin II and consequently:

- Decrease vasoconstriction
- Decrease aldosterone (and prevent an increase in ECF volume).

Adrenal insufficiency is a condition where the adrenal glands fail to secrete the required hormone levels. It normally has a non-specific presentation unless the patient is having an acute adrenal crisis, which is typically life threatening. On investigation, the patient may have abnormally high potassium levels (hyperkalaemia) and low sodium levels (hyponatraemia). These findings result from reduced aldosterone secretion and resultant renal Na^+ wasting and reduced K^+ excretion.

Aldosterone

Aldosterone is synthesized by zona glomerulosa cells in the adrenal cortex. Its release (Fig. 3.16) is controlled by:

- Angiotensin II.
- ECF volume: if circulating Na^+ falls, effective circulating volume also falls. This stimulates aldosterone release via the RAA system.

- Increased sympathetic innervation: a fall in ECF volume results in a fall in blood pressure. This is detected by baroreceptors in carotid arteries and causes increased sympathetic activity. Granular cells of the JGA are innervated by the sympathetic system, so an increase in sympathetic activity leads to an increase in renin release. The process is mediated by β-adrenergic receptors.
- The wall tension in afferent arterioles falls: decreased ECF volume reduces blood pressure, which in turn decreases perfusion pressure to the kidneys. Changes in the blood pressure decrease wall tension at granular cells, which stimulates renin release.
- Decreased Na^+ to the macula densa: if less NaCl reaches the macula densa, the macula densa is stimulated to secrete the prostaglandin PGI_2. This acts on the granular cells to cause renin release.

Fig. 3.16 Factors causing aldosterone release and the effects of aldosterone. ECF, extracellular fluid.

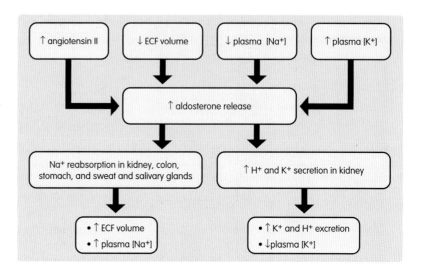

- Na^+ concentration: via direct aldosterone release from the adrenal cortex, as well as through the RAA system.
- K^+ concentration: a rise in circulating K^+ stimulates direct release of aldosterone from the adrenal cortex. This returns K^+ to normal by increasing distal tubular secretion of K^+.

Aldosterone primarily regulates sodium concentration. It acts within cells to:

- Promote Na^+ reabsorption in the kidney, colon, gastric glands and sweat and salivary gland ducts
- Promote K^+ and H^+ secretion by the kidney.

Factors affecting Na^+ reabsorption

Starling's forces in the proximal tubule

The amount of Na^+ and water reabsorbed into the peritubular capillaries from the proximal tubule depends on the rate and amount of uptake from the lateral intercellular spaces into the capillaries.

Changes in the body fluid volume alters plasma hydrostatic and oncotic pressure, for example, increased NaCl intake is mirrored by a rise in ECF volume. This in turn increases hydrostatic pressure and decreases oncotic pressure, so NaCl and water reabsorption by the proximal tubule cells decreases.

Sympathetic drive from the renal nerves

The arterial baroreceptors regulate renal sympathetic nerve activity, for example, a fall in ECF volume decreases blood pressure, which is sensed by baro-

receptors, and results in an increase in sympathetic activity. This stimulates Na^+ retention and an increase in peripheral resistance, thus restoring ECF volume and blood pressure.

A rise in sympathetic nerve activity to the kidney stimulates renin release either directly or as a result of renal vasoconstriction (this activates the JGA). Catecholamines from sympathetic nerve endings also stimulate Na^+ reabsorption by the proximal tubule, but it is unclear if this is a direct effect or secondary to altered peritubular forces.

Prostaglandins

A decrease in the effective circulating volume stimulates cortical prostaglandin (PG) synthesis. In the kidney, PG synthesis occurs in the:

- Cortex (arterioles and glomeruli)
- Medullary interstitial cells
- Collecting duct epithelial cells.

Several prostaglandins exist: PGE_2 (medullary), PGI_2 (cortical), $PGF_{2\alpha}$, PGD_2 and thromboxane A_2 (TXA_2). The main functions of each are as follows:

- PGE_2, PGI_2: vasodilators, preventing excessive vasoconstriction.
- PGI_2 (prostacyclin): renin release.
- PGE_2 (medullary): promotes water (diuretic) and sodium (natriuretic) excretion within the collecting tubules and thus overrides the antidiuretic action of ADH. PGE_2 protects the medullary tubule cells from excessive hypoxia when the ECF volume decreases.

- TXA_2: a vasoconstrictor, which is synthesized after repeated kidney damage (e.g. ureteral obstruction). It reduces the amount of blood available for filtration by a poorly functioning kidney.

Atrial natriuretic peptide (ANP)

ANP is a peptide produced by cardiac atrial cells in response to an increase in ECF volume. It is found in the atrial cells and released into the plasma. ANP binds to specific cell surface receptors, resulting in increased cyclic guanosine monosulphate (cGMP). ANP acts to:

- Inhibit Na^+/K^+ ATPase and close Na^+ channels of the collecting ducts, reducing Na^+ reabsorption. Na^+ reabsorption is also reduced in the proximal tubules. Thus, Na^+ and water excretion by the kidney is increased
- Vasodilate afferent arterioles, thereby increasing GFR
- Inhibit aldosterone secretion
- Inhibit ADH release
- Decrease renin release.

Dopamine

This is synthesized by the proximal tubule cells and:

- Inhibits Na^+/K^+ ATPase and Na^+/H^+ antiport, thereby decreasing tubular Na^+ transport
- Increases Na^+ excretion (natriuresis)
- Causes vasodilation.

Kinins

Kininogens are cleaved by the enzyme kallikrein to form kinins. The effects of kinins are similar to PGs and include:

- Vasodilation
- Inhibition of ADH release
- Increased Na^+ excretion.

Natriuretic hormone

This hormone inhibits the Na^+/K^+ ATPase enzyme and is thought to be produced by the hypothalamus. Figure 3.17 summarizes the mechanisms involved in the regulation of body fluid.

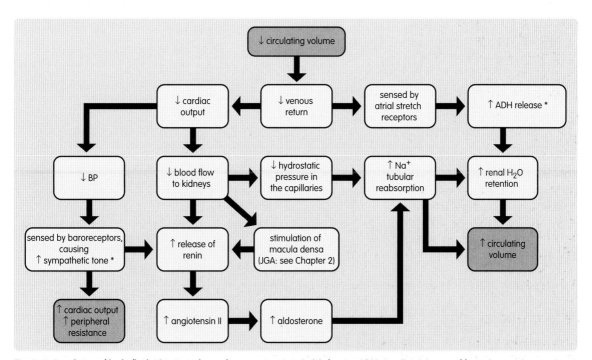

Fig. 3.17 Regulation of body fluid. JGA, juxtaglomerular apparatus. Asterix (*) denotes ADH secretion is increased by an increase in sympathetic tone.

REGULATION OF BODY FLUID pH

Body fluid pH is tightly controlled because most enzyme reactions are sensitive to pH changes.

- Normal pH range is 7.35–7.45
- Normal H^+ concentration is 35–45 nmol/L.

Buffers

Definition

A buffer is a mixture of a weak acid (HA) and a conjugate base. It undergoes minimal pH change when either an acid or a base is added to it:

$$HA \rightleftharpoons H^+ \text{ (acid)} + A^- \text{ (conjugate base)}$$

It can also be a mixture of a weak base (BH) and conjugate acid:

$$BH \rightleftharpoons H^+ \text{ (conjugate acid)} + B^- \text{ (base)}$$

For example, if there is an increase in H^+, the equations above shift to the left so that the extra H^+ combines with the buffer and the H^+ concentration in the body falls.

The kidneys act together with the lungs and buffer systems to minimize any changes in plasma $[H^+]$.

pK values and equilibrium constants

The equations below demonstrate the equilibrium constants in terms of conjugate acids and bases, proton donators, and acceptors.

$$HA \rightleftharpoons H^+ + A^-$$

Equation 1. At equilibrium:

$$k = \frac{[H^+][A^-]}{[HA]}$$

$$\therefore [H^+] = \frac{k[HA]}{[A^-]}$$

$$= \frac{k \, [acid]}{[base]}$$

Equation 2:

$$pH = -\log [H^+]$$

$$= \frac{\log 1}{[H^+]}$$

$$pK = -\log k$$

$$= \frac{\log 1}{k}$$

Equation 3. Combining equations 1 and 2 (the Henderson–Hasselbalch equation).

$$pH = pK + \frac{\log [base]}{[acid]}$$

Physiological buffers

There are several buffer systems in the different body compartments (Fig. 3.18), of which the most important is the bicarbonate buffer system.

Bicarbonate buffer system

The bicarbonate buffer system is important in all body fluids. CO_2 and H_2O combine to form carbonic acid (H_2CO_3) in the presence of the enzyme carbonic anhydrase (CA). The H_2CO_3 then dissociates spontaneously to form bicarbonate ions (HCO_3^-) and H^+. This is summarized in the equation below:

$$CO_2 + H_2O \underset{\xrightarrow{\text{anhydrase}}}{\overset{\text{carbonic}}{\rightleftharpoons}} H_2CO_3 \rightleftharpoons H^+ + HCO_3^-$$

CO_2 concentration is regulated by the lungs and HCO_3^- concentration is regulated by the kidneys. Therefore, pH regulation depends equally on both these organs. Substituting this equation in the Henderson–Hasselbalch equation, we get:

Fig. 3.18 Buffer systems in different body compartments

Buffer systems	Blood	ECF and CSF	ICF
HCO_3^-/CO_2	✓	✓	✓
haemoglobin	✓		
plasma proteins	✓		
phosphate	✓	✓	✓
organic phosphate			✓
proteins		✓	✓

Note: CSF, cerebrospinal fluid; ECF, extracellular fluid; ICF, intracellular fluid

$$pH = pK + \log \frac{[HCO_3^-]}{[H_2CO_3]}$$

$[H_2CO_3]$ is determined by dissolved CO_2:

$[H_2CO_3] = 0.23 \times pCO_2$ (0.23 is the CO_2 solubility coefficient at 37 °C; pCO_2 is the pressure of CO_2 in the lungs)

Therefore, $pH = \dfrac{pK + \log[HCO_3^-]}{0.23 \times pCO_2}$

Normal values are:

- $[HCO_3^-]$: 20–30 mmol/L
- pCO_2: 4.4–5.3 kPa
- pK of HCO_3^-/pCO_2 system: 6.1.

Therefore pH = 7.4. In summary:

$$pH \propto \frac{HCO_3^-}{pCO_2}$$

Renal regulation of plasma HCO_3^-

H^+ is produced during metabolism, which stimulates CO_2 production:

$$H^+ + HCO_3^- \rightleftharpoons H_2CO_3 \rightleftharpoons H_2O + CO_2$$

CO_2 is exhaled by the lungs. The kidneys retain HCO_3^- and make more HCO_3^-.

The concentration of HCO_3^- in the plasma filtered by the kidney is 25 mmol/L. HCO_3^- is re-absorbed by the kidney using a T_m-dependent mechanism (Fig. 3.19). The T_m is similar to the amount of HCO_3^- filtered at a normal plasma concentration. If plasma HCO_3^- increases, T_m is exceeded

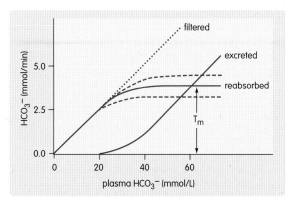

Fig. 3.19 How HCO_3^- ions are handled by the kidney. HCO_3^- absorption is dependent on H^+ secretion into the tubule. This dependency causes the T_m for HCO_3^- absorption to vary. The limits of the T_m variability are illustrated by the dotted lines on the graph.

and HCO_3^- is excreted until the plasma level returns to normal. Figure 3.19 illustrates the way in which HCO_3^- is handled by the kidney.

Ninety per cent of HCO_3^- is absorbed in the proximal tubule (see Chapter 2).

HCO_3^- reabsorption

In the proximal tubule: the lumen
HCO_3^- reacts with H^+ (delivered into the lumen via an antiport process coupled with Na^+) to give H_2CO_3. H_2CO_3 dissociates into H_2O and CO_2, catalysed by the enzyme CA (present in the brush border of luminal cells). CA inhibitors suppress H^+ secretion, leading to a fall in Na^+ and HCO_3^- absorption, and thus act as a weak diuretic.

In the proximal tubule: the tubular cells
H_2O and CO_2 enter the tubular cells and re-form H_2CO_3, catalysed by CA. H_2CO_3 again dissociates into:

- H^+, which is secreted into the lumen
- HCO_3^-, which enters the plasma via the peritubular fluid (see also Chapter 2).

Some HCO_3^- couples with luminal Cl^- so that HCO_3^- is secreted into the lumen and Cl^- is absorbed.

In the distal tubule
This involves intercalated cells. Secreted H^+ and luminal HCO_3^- are present but CA is limited. Therefore little CO_2 and H_2O are produced, so less HCO_3^- is absorbed. H^+ ions are secreted across into the lumen by H^+ ATPase and H^+/K^+ ATPase (pumps H^+ out and K^+ in).

Conversion of alkaline phosphate to acid phosphate – luminal buffer

Alkaline phosphate Na_2HPO_4 and acid phosphate NaH_2PO_4 are present in the plasma in the ratio of 4:1. Both are filtered at the glomerulus. Alkaline phosphate is converted to acid phosphate, mainly in the distal tubule but also in the proximal tubule (Fig. 3.20). This generates HCO_3^- for the plasma.

Ammonia secretion – luminal buffer

Deamination of glutamine in the proximal tubule produces ammonium ions (NH_4^+) (see Fig. 3.20). Although the liver can metabolize NH_4^+ to urea, it is only by secretion of NH_4^+ in the kidney that HCO_3^- can be regenerated to act as a buffer in the plasma.

Fig. 3.20 Conversion of alkaline phosphate to acid phosphate in the tubule lumen. This conversion liberates free sodium, which is transported into the tubule cell by an Na^+/H^+ antiporter, causing H^+ secretion into the lumen and increased HCO_3^- reabsorption by the tubule cells. CA, carbonic anhydrase.

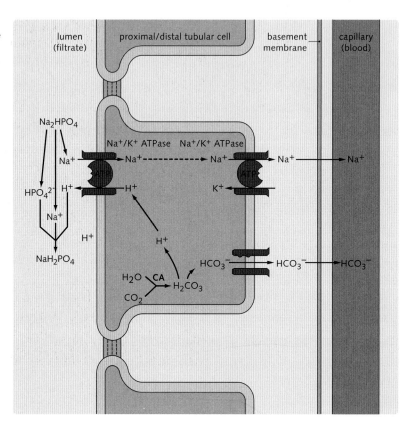

However, 50% of NH_4^+ secreted into the proximal tubule is reabsorbed by the thick ascending limb of the loop of Henle and accumulates in the cells of the medullary interstitium (see Fig. 3.22). Figure 3.21 illustrates the secretion and handling of ammonia (NH_3) and Fig. 3.22 shows NH_3 and NH_4^+ handling by the nephrons.

Acidosis increases NH_4^+ excretion because:

- Acidosis stimulates enzymes that deaminate glutamine, thereby increasing NH_4^+ synthesis.
- Increased H^+ secretion results in NH_3 production, which in turn results in increased NH_4^+ in the collecting tubules. The conversion of NH_3 to NH_4^+ maintains a gradient for NH_3 secretion. In this way, excess NH_3/NH_4^+ is removed from the medulla.

Acid–base disturbances

There are four main types:

1. Respiratory acidosis
2. Respiratory alkalosis
3. Metabolic (non-respiratory origin) acidosis
4. Metabolic alkalosis.

Metabolic disturbances result from changes in cellular metabolism or diet, so are independent of pCO_2 changes. If the body fluid pH alters, the buffering system mechanism is activated. Thus, overall, there might be very little change in arterial pH despite acid–base imbalance. A change in the arterial pH results in a change in the pH of body cells, which adversely affects many cellular processes.

The Davenport diagram is a graph of the plasma HCO_3^- versus plasma pH, used to classify acid–base disturbances (Fig. 3.23).

Compensation and correction

- Compensation is the restoration of normal pH even when acid–base imbalance is still present
- Correction is the restoration of both the pH and acid–base imbalance to normal:

$$H_2O + CO_2 \rightleftharpoons H_2CO_3 \rightleftharpoons H^+ + HCO_3^-$$

$$pH \propto \frac{HCO_3^-}{pCO_2}$$

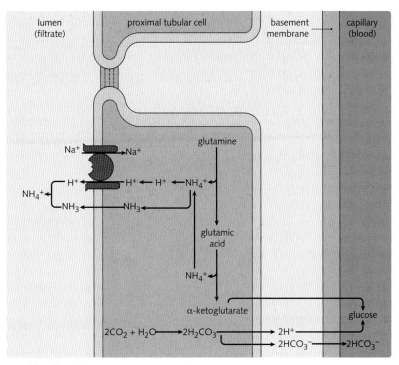

Fig. 3.21 Renal secretion and handling of NH_3.

Therefore, if two variables (e.g. pH and pCO_2) are known, $[HCO_3^-]$ can be calculated.

Arterial blood gases (ABGs) measure the pH, pO_2 and pCO_2 in an arterial blood sample. This can be used to diagnose an acid–base imbalance. For example, if pH = 7.2 and pCO_2 is 9.3 kPa, by looking at Figure 3.23 it can be seen that $[HCO_3^-]$ will be raised. This corresponds to a respiratory acidosis.

Examples of acid–base disturbances

Respiratory acidosis

The causes of respiratory acidosis are:

- Chronic obstructive pulmonary disease (COPD)
- Obstruction of the airway (e.g. tumour, foreign body)
- Mechanical chest injuries

- Severe asthma
- Drugs: general anaesthetic, morphine, barbiturates (respiratory centre depressant)
- Injuries and infections to the respiratory centre in the brainstem.

ABG results show $pCO_2 > 6.0$ kPa and decreased pH. Clinically, the respiratory system cannot remove enough CO_2, so CO_2 increases together with pCO_2. Therefore the following equation is shifted to the right:

$$\xrightarrow{\hspace{3cm}}$$

$$CO_2 + H_2O \rightleftharpoons H_2CO_3 \rightleftharpoons H^+ + HCO_3^-$$

This results in elevated $[H^+]$ and $[HCO_3^-]$. The extra H^+ results in increased H^+ secretion and increased HCO_3^- reabsorption. This restores pH, acting as a compensatory response. The acid–base disturbance is not corrected because the pCO_2 and $[HCO_3^-]$ are

Fig. 3.22 Handling of NH$_3$ and NH$_4^+$ by nephrons.

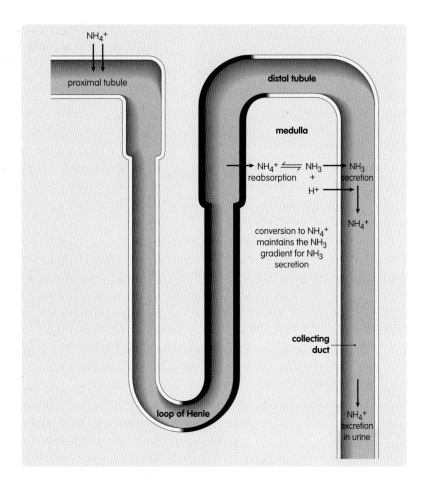

Fig. 3.23 Acid and base disturbances with compensatory changes demonstrated on the Davenport diagram.

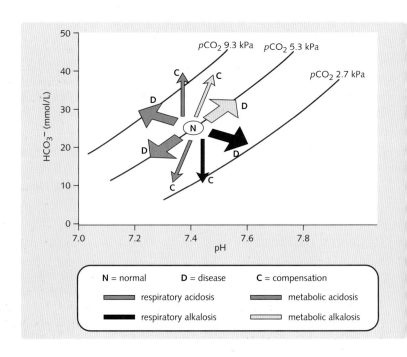

still high. Correction requires hyperventilation to decrease pCO_2.

Figure 3.23 illustrates acid–base disturbances with compensatory changes.

Respiratory alkalosis

The causes of respiratory alkalosis are:

- Decreased pO_2, which is detected by chemoreceptors in the carotid body, resulting in hyperventilation and decreased pCO_2
- High altitude
- Fever
- Brainstem damage resulting in hyperventilation
- Hysterical overbreathing.

The ABG results show a $pCO_2 < 4.7$ kPa and an elevated pH. Clinically, too much CO_2 is removed by the respiratory system. Therefore the following equation is shifted to the left:

$$CO_2 + H_2O \rightleftharpoons H_2CO_3 \rightleftharpoons H^+ + HCO_3^-$$

This causes [H$^+$] to fall and hence an increased pH and a slight decrease in [HCO$_3^-$]. The compensatory response involves reduced H$^+$ secretion, increased HCO$_3^-$ excretion and decreased HCO$_3^-$ reabsorption, thus restoring pH. Correction involves rectification of the underlying respiratory defect.

A primary decrease in plasma bicarbonate and a slight reduction in pH indicate a metabolic acidosis. This may be caused by failure of the kidneys to excrete H$^+$ or reabsorb HCO$_3$. This may be caused by renal tubular acidosis types I, II and IV. It is important to note that the acidosis refers to the plasma pH, not that of the tubular fluid and that the urine can be alkaline. Alkali is usually administered to correct the acidosis.

Metabolic acidosis

The causes of metabolic acidosis are:

- Ingestion of acids (H$^+$)
- Excess metabolic production of H$^+$ (e.g. lactate acidosis, diabetic ketoacidosis)
- Loss of HCO$_3^-$ (e.g. severe diarrhoea, drainage from fistulae)
- Renal disease (failure to excrete H$^+$).

ABG results show a normal pCO_2 and decreased pH. There is an increase in [H$^+$]. Therefore, the following equation is shifted to the left:

$$CO_2 + H_2O \rightleftharpoons H_2CO_3 \rightleftharpoons H^+ + HCO_3^-$$

Consequently, [HCO$_3^-$] falls as it is used to 'mop up' the excess H$^+$ ions.

The decreased pH stimulates respiration to cause hyperventilation. This respiratory compensation decreases pCO_2 and returns the pH to normal, although HCO$_3^-$ falls further. The fall in HCO$_3^-$ hinders the compensatory response of the kidneys, which is to increase HCO$_3^-$ reabsorption and produce titratable acid.

The anion gap represents the difference between plasma anions and cations and represents un-accounted anions (e.g. phosphates, ketones, lactate):

$$\text{Anion gap} = ([K^+] + [Na^+]) - ([Cl^-] + [HCO_3^-])$$

The normal range is 8–16 mmol/L. Changes in the anion gap help define the cause of a metabolic acidosis. Metabolic acidosis due to diarrhoea or renal tubular acidosis does not alter the anion gap. Acidosis caused by renal failure, diabetes or lactic acidosis increases the anion gap.

Metabolic alkalosis

The causes of metabolic alkalosis are:

- Loss of acid (e.g. vomiting, diarrhoea)
- Ingestion of alkali (e.g. antacid ingestion)
- Depleted ECF (e.g. haemorrhage, burns, excess diuretic use, contraction alkalosis).

ABG results show a normal pCO_2 and an elevated pH because of a rise in plasma [HCO$_3^-$]. Therefore, the following equation is shifted to the right:

$$CO_2 + H_2O \rightleftharpoons H_2CO_3 \rightleftharpoons H^+ + HCO_3^- \ H^+ + OH^- \rightarrow H_2O$$

Consequently, [HCO$_3^-$] is increased.

Respiratory compensation occurs. The increase in pH acts on chemoreceptors, which reduce the ventilatory rate and so increase pCO_2. The equation therefore shifts to the right and the pH returns to normal, but HCO$_3^-$ increases further. This hinders correction (see Fig. 3.23).

Fig. 3.24 Summary of acid–base disturbances and compensatory mechanisms

Acid–base disturbance	pH	pCO_2	HCO_3^-	Clinical cause	Compensation
respiratory acidosis	↓	↑	↑	severe asthma; COPD	metabolic ($\uparrow HCO_3^-$)
respiratory alkalosis	↑	↓	↓	hyperventilation	metabolic ($\downarrow HCO_3^-$)
metabolic acidosis	↓	normal	↓	diabetic ketoacidosis; chronic renal failure	respiratory ($\downarrow pCO_2$)
metabolic alkalosis	↑	normal	↑	vomiting	respiratory ($\uparrow pCO_2$)

Figure 3.24 summarizes acid–base disturbances.

REGULATION OF CALCIUM AND PHOSPHATE

Calcium (Ca^{2+})

Ca^{2+} is present mainly in bone but has an important extraskeletal function. The threshold potential of cell membranes of nerve and muscle for action potentials varies inversely with plasma calcium concentration. Thus it is important to keep calcium levels constant.

Calcium exists in two forms in the plasma:

1. Ionized Ca^{2+}, which is physiologically more important (normal concentration: 1.25 mmol/L).
2. Ca^{2+} bound to protein – mainly albumin (normal concentration: 1.25 mmol/L).

Ca^{2+} concentrations are:

- Total plasma Ca^{2+}: 2.2–2.6 mmol/L
- ECF Ca^{2+}: 1.25 mmol/L
- Interstitial fluid total Ca^{2+}: 1.25 mmol/L
- Intracellular Ca^{2+}: 0.0001 mmol/L; found in smooth endothelial reticulum and mitochondria, complexed with calmodulin.

It is important to maintain a low intracellular Ca^{2+}.

Clinical features and causes of Ca^{2+} disturbances

Hypocalcaemia
Causes are:

- Hypoparathyroidism
- Rickets and osteomalacia (low vitamin D)
- Hypomagnesaemia
- Pancreatitis
- Alkalosis, which reduces the amount of H^+ available to bind to protein, so more Ca^{2+} can bind to protein. This results in decreased ionized Ca^{2+}, although total Ca^{2+} remains the same
- Chronic renal failure, due to hyperphosphataemia (if PO_4^{3-} rises, Ca^{2+} must fall proportionally) and low levels of activated vitamin D.

Decreased Ca^{2+} results in tetany with convulsions, hand and feet muscle cramps (leading to paralysis) and cardiac arrhythmias.

Hypercalcaemia
Causes of hypercalcaemia are:

- Primary hyperparathyroidism
- Sudden acidosis, resulting in the release of bound calcium, which becomes ionized Ca^{2+}
- Increased intestinal absorption due to excess vitamin D or ingestion of calcium (milk–alkali syndrome)

- Bone destruction resulting in increased Ca^{2+} release from bone – usually caused by secondary deposits from malignancy or myeloma
- Production of humoral hypercalcaemic agents by tumours
- Granulomatous disease (sarcoid)
- Drugs, e.g. thiazides
- Tertiary hyperparathyroidism in chronic renal failure
- Hypermagnesaemia.

Symptoms and signs of hypercalcaemia are:

- Renal calculi
- Behaviour disturbance (because of the effects on higher cerebral functions)
- Constipation due to decreased intestinal mobility
- Renal damage
- Calcification outside the skeletal system
- Polyuria
- Polydipsia.

Ca^{2+} transport by the kidney

Only ionized Ca^{2+} is filtered through the glomerulus (approximately 50% plasma Ca^{2+}). Reabsorption proceeds as follows:

- Proximal tubule: 70% is reabsorbed by diffusion, Ca^{2+}-activated ATPase and the Ca^{2+}/Na^+ counter-transport system.
- Thick ascending loop of Henle: 20–25% is reabsorbed passively.
- Distal convoluted tubule: 5–10% is reabsorbed against an electrochemical gradient.
- Collecting tubule: less than 0.5% is reabsorbed against an electrochemical gradient.

Calcium and phosphate homeostasis

Ca^{2+} and PO_4^{3-} concentrations are inversely proportional.

$$[Ca^{2+}] \times [PO_4^{3-}] = constant$$

Therefore, a rise in Ca^{2+} leads to a decrease in PO_4^{3-}, whereas a fall in Ca^{2+} stimulates an increase in PO_4^{3-} concentration, and vice versa.

Ca^{2+} and PO_4^{3-} enter the ECF via the intestine (diet) and bone stores. They leave the ECF via the kidneys (urine) and move into the bone.

Parathyroid hormone (PTH), vitamin D and calcitonin regulate Ca^{2+} and PO_4^{3-}.

PTH

PTH is a polypeptide secreted by the parathyroid gland when there is a fall in plasma Ca^{2+}. PO_4^{3-} also affects PTH release, both directly and secondary to changes in Ca^{2+} levels. Figure 3.25 illustrates mechanisms of Ca^{2+} and PO_4^{3-} homeostasis. Vitamin D can also affect PTH release because it alters sensitivity of the parathyroid gland to Ca^{2+}.

Vitamin D

Vitamin D refers to a group of closely related sterols obtained from the diet or by the action of ultraviolet light on certain provitamins. It is metabolized to 1,25-dihydroxycholecalciferol by the liver and kidney. This causes an increase in Ca^{2+} and PO_4^{3-} by:

- Enhancing intestinal absorption of Ca^{2+}
- Increasing Ca^{2+} release from bone
- Decreasing Ca^{2+} and PO_4^{3-} excretion.

Calcitonin

Calcitonin is a peptide produced by the parafollicular cells of the thyroid. It reduces Ca^{2+} release from bone causing a decrease in ECF Ca^{2+} concentration.

Phosphate

Phosphate is present in the plasma and interstitial fluid as:

- 'Acid' phosphate $H_2PO_4^-$
- 'Alkaline' phosphate HPO_4^{3-}.

The proportion of the two forms depends on plasma pH. In cells, both inorganic forms (acid phosphate and alkaline phosphate) and organic forms (ATP, ADP and cAMP) are found. Plasma phosphate concentration is 0.8–1.3 mmol/L.

The kidney handles PO_4^{3-} as follows:

- Alkaline phosphate and acid phosphate are filtered by the glomerulus in a ratio of 4:1. Alkaline phosphate is converted to acid phosphate in the tubule as a result of H^+ secretion (see Fig. 3.20).
- 95% of the filtered PO_4^{3-} is reabsorbed in the early proximal tubule.
- Renal PO_4^{3-} excretion is increased by PTH, which is the only hormone to regulate phosphate transport.

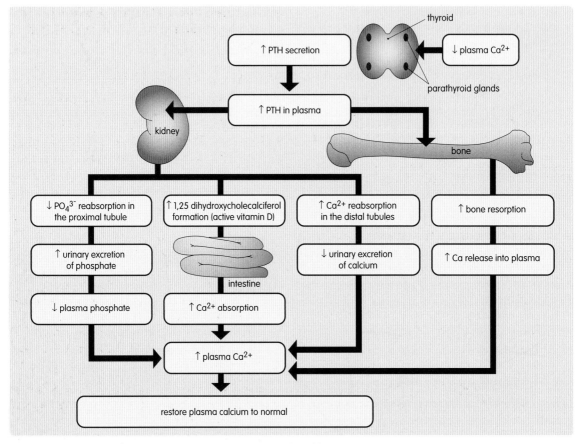

Fig. 3.25 Mechanisms of Ca^{2+} and phosphate homoeostasis. PTH, parathyroid hormone.

REGULATION OF POTASSIUM AND MAGNESIUM

Potassium

Potassium (K^+) is the main intracellular cation. The intracellular and extracellular [K^+] is very important in the function of excitable tissues (e.g. nerves and muscles) as it determines the resting potentials of these tissues. Therefore, a constant [K^+] is critical for survival. Concentration is as follows:

- Total body K^+: 3–4 mmol/L
- Intracellular fluid (ICF) K^+: 98%; 150–160 mmol/L
- Extracellular fluid (ECF) K^+: 2%; 4–5 mmol/L.

- If extracellular [K^+] rises, the resting membrane potential is decreased (i.e. depolarized).
- If extracellular [K^+] falls, the resting membrane potential is increased (i.e. hyperpolarized).

Clinical features and causes of K^+ disturbances

Hypokalaemia

Causes of a decreased K^+ concentration are:

- Vomiting
- Diarrhoea

- Diuretics
- Excess insulin (e.g. Cushing's syndrome, steroids)
- Renal tubular acidosis.

Hypokalaemia is asymptomatic until K^+ concentration falls below 2–2.5 mmol/L. The low K^+ concentration results in a decreased resting potential (more negative) so the nerve and muscle cells become hyperpolarized. This means that cells are less sensitive to depolarizing stimuli and therefore less excitable, so fewer action potentials are generated and paralysis ensues. Clinical effects of hypokalaemia are:

- Muscle weakness, cramps and tetany, which starts in the lower extremities and progresses upwards (death is usually by paralysis of respiratory muscles)
- Impaired liver conversion of glucose to glycogen
- Vasoconstriction and cardiac arrhythmias
- Impaired ADH action, causing thirst and polyuria and no concentration of urine
- Metabolic alkalosis due to an increase in intracellular H^+ concentration.

Treatment involves treating the underlying cause, and calculated oral or intravenous administration of potassium salt may be required.

Hyperkalaemia

Causes of an increased K^+ concentration are:

- Ingestion of K^+
- Metabolic acidosis (diabetes mellitus)
- Insulin deficiency (i.e. Addison's disease)
- Excess cell breakdown (e.g. after cytotoxic cancer therapy)
- Renal failure.

Hyperkalaemia is asymptomatic until $K^+ > 6.5$ mmol/L. The increased K^+ concentration results in cell depolarization and increased excitability. The resting potential might be above the threshold potential, so cells cannot repolarize after an action potential, leading to paralysis. Death results from cardiac arrest due to the effects of hyperkalaemia on cardiac conduction. Fatal arrhythmias can occur when $K^+ > 7$ mmol/L.
  Treatment involves:

- Dextrose and insulin to drive K^+ into cells
- HCO_3^- to correct acidosis by stimulating K^+ entry into cells
- Calcium salts to protect excitable tissues (of heart) against toxic effects of K^+

- K^+ removal from body using loop diuretics, exchange resins (i.e. calcium resonium), and dialysis.

K^+ transport by the kidney

K^+ is filtered freely in the glomerulus. The proximal tubule reabsorbs 80–90%:

- Passively
- Through tight junctions (paracellular movement)
- Via a concentration gradient.

In the distal tubule:

- K^+ reabsorption and leakage back are approximately equal in the early distal tubule
- The late distal tubule and collecting ducts secrete K^+ into the urinary filtrate (passively via an electrochemical gradient) according to the body's needs – increased cellular K^+ concentration results in increased secretion and vice versa.

Changes in the distal tubular lumen also influence the rate of K^+ secretion. Figure 3.26 illustrates K^+ transport in the kidney.
  ADH stimulates the secretion of K^+ by the collecting ducts by enhancing Na^+ reabsorption. Aldosterone increases K^+ secretion. Increased plasma K^+ concentration stimulates aldosterone production by the adrenal cortex, so plasma aldosterone concentration rises. This in turn increases K^+ secretion and therefore K^+ excretion.

Magnesium

Magnesium (Mg^{2+}) is an intracellular cation that:

- Controls mitochondrial oxidative metabolism and so regulates energy production
- Is vital for protein synthesis.
- Regulates K^+ and Ca^{2+} channels in cell membranes.

The plasma concentration of magnesium is 2.12–2.65 mmol/L; about 20% is protein bound. Total body magnesium is 28g, of which:

- 55% is in bone
- 40% is in ICF
- Up to 10% is in plasma at any one time
- 0.6% is in ECF.

Fig. 3.26 Potassium transport in the kidney.

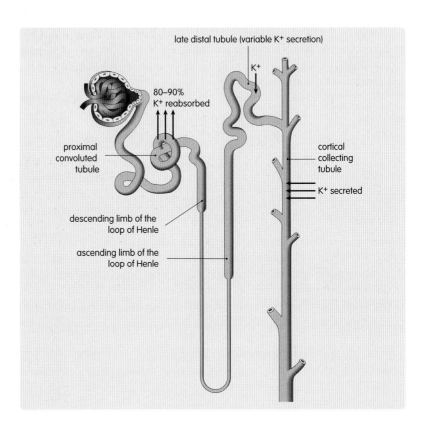

late distal tubule (variable K⁺ secretion)

80–90% K⁺ reabsorbed

proximal convoluted tubule

cortical collecting tubule

K⁺ secreted

descending limb of the loop of Henle

ascending limb of the loop of Henle

Clinical features and causes of Mg²⁺ disturbances

Hypomagnesaemia

Causes are:

- Decreased intake
- Diarrhoea
- Absorption disorder including fat absorption defects
- Renal wasting – intrinsic (Bartter's syndrome), extrinsic (diuretics, e.g. thiazides).

Clinical features are non-specific. A fall in Mg²⁺ is followed by a decreased Ca²⁺, but the mechanism for this is unknown.

Renal handling of Mg²⁺

- In the glomerulus ionized Mg²⁺ (75% of total Mg²⁺) is filtered
- 15% is reabsorbed in the proximal tubule
- 60% is reabsorbed in the thick ascending loop of Henle – the Na⁺/K⁺/Cl⁻ co-transporter system enables Mg²⁺ absorption through the paracellular route. An Na⁺/Mg²⁺ antiport and Mg²⁺ ATPase transport system also exists

- Up to 5% is reabsorbed in the distal convoluted tubule
- 0.5% is reabsorbed in the collecting tubule.

Regulation of Mg²⁺

The T_m for Mg²⁺ absorption is equal to the concentration of Mg²⁺ filtered. Therefore, an increase in Mg²⁺ results in increased filtering, which therefore exceeds the T_m, resulting in increased excretion.

There is intrinsic regulation by cells of the thick ascending loop of Henle – if Mg²⁺ decreases, cell transport of Mg²⁺ increases. PTH increases reabsorption of Mg²⁺ in the thick ascending loop of Henle.

REGULATION OF ERYTHROPOIESIS

Erythropoietin (EPO) is a glycoprotein hormone involved in erythrocyte production by the bone marrow. Although it is produced in the liver, the main source of EPO (over 80%) is the kidney (renal tubulo-interstitial cells). The kidneys secrete EPO in response to a low tissue oxygen tension. This occurs in hypoxia and anaemia, and is an attempt to increase the number of circulating red blood cells and therefore improve tissue oxygen delivery. This response is thought to be mediated by PG, which stimulates the intrarenal synthesis of EPO. EPO-sensitive stem cells are converted into proerythroblasts and then into red blood cells in the bone marrow.

Patients with chronic renal failure often have defective EPO production, leading to normocytic normochromic anaemia. This can be treated by administration of exogenous (synthetic) EPO, which is produced using recombinant DNA technology. Typically subcutaneous or intravenous injections up to three times a week at a dose of 30–50 U/kg are required to reach a haemoglobin (Hb) count of 10–12 g/dL and eliminate the need for blood transfusions.

Iron deficiency is the most common cause of failure in EPO treatment, and is corrected with oral or intravenous supplements. Other reasons for failure to respond include bleeding, malignancy, hyperparathyroidism, inadequate dialysis, inflammation and infection.

The complications of treatment are thrombotic complication, hypertension and fitting. These are associated with rapid increases in Hb concentration and haematocrit.

Objectives

By the end of the chapter you should be able to:

- Compare and contrast unilateral and bilateral renal agenesis. Explain what causes renal agenesis
- Understand the genetics of adult polycystic kidney disease. Discuss how the prognosis in adult polycystic kidney disease differs from that in childhood polycystic kidney disease
- Classify glomerular disease
- Discuss the main clinical syndromes associated with glomerular disease, giving examples of typical clinical manifestations
- Explain how nephritic syndrome (i.e. acute nephritis) differs from nephrotic syndrome
- Outline the causes of acute tubular nephritis
- Discuss the incidence, presentation and diagnosis of urinary tract infections
- Discuss the aetiology, predisposing factors and appearance of the kidney in acute and chronic pyelonephritis
- Outline the changes seen in the renal vasculature in hypertension. Describe the two main types of hypertension
- Describe the aetiology and management of renal artery stenosis
- Explain the causes of haemolytic uraemic syndrome
- Discuss renal cell carcinoma, noting its incidence, the age group affected, predisposing factors, presentation and morphology
- Describe Wilms' tumour
- Explain the compensatory mechanisms that occur in the kidney in heart failure
- Outline the different types of shock and their effects on renal physiology
- Describe which immune disorders affect the kidney
- Discuss the site and mechanism of action, uses and side-effects of the different classes of diuretics
- Outline the role of angiotensin-converting enzyme inhibitors in the treatment of hypertension, indicating their mechanisms of action and side-effects
- Be able to discuss the different types of renal replacement therapy.

CONGENITAL ABNORMALITIES OF THE KIDNEY

Congenital structural abnormalities can develop within the kidney, as described below.

Agenesis of the kidney

Absence (agenesis) of the kidney can be unilateral or bilateral. Unilateral agenesis occurs in 1 in 1000 of the population. Agenesis occurs if the collecting system (from the ureteric buds) fails to fuse with the nephrons (from the metanephric mesoderm). The remaining kidney gradually hypertrophies but may also be abnormal with malrotation, ectopia or hydronephrosis. Renal function may still be normal. There is risk of infection and trauma to the solitary kidney. This disorder is associated with other developmental abnormalities such as absent testes or ovaries, spina bifida and congenital heart disease. Bilateral agenesis occurs in less than 1 in 3000 pregnancies and is incompatible with life. It is also known as Potter's syndrome, which is associated with pulmonary hypoplasia and oligohydramnios in utero. There is no treatment.

Potter's syndrome, or bilateral agenesis, is characterized by renal agenesis, leading to oligohydramnios and hypoplastic lungs. The infant has low-set ears, a flattened nose and wide-set eyes.

Hypoplasia

The kidneys develop inadequately and are consequently smaller than average. This is a rare disorder, affecting one or both kidneys, which are prone to infection and stone formation. It may also cause secondary hypertension.

Ectopic kidney

The incidence of ectopic kidney is 1 in 800. The kidney does not ascend fully into the abdomen, so remains lower than usual (if it remains in the pelvis, it is called a 'pelvic kidney'). It is usually unilateral and, the lower the kidney, the more abnormal it is. As a result of the abnormal positioning, the ureters can be obstructed by neighbouring structures, leading to obstructive uropathy, infection and stone formation. This disorder can also cause obstruction during birth.

Horseshoe kidney

The incidence of horseshoe kidney, a type of ectopic kidney, is between 1 in 600 and 1 in 1800, and is more common in boys than girls. The two kidneys fuse across the midline, usually at their lower poles, by renal tissue or a fibrous band (Fig. 4.1). The horseshoe kidney is usually lower than normal because the inferior mesenteric artery limits its ascent. It can also be malrotated and is prone to reflux, obstruction, infection and stone formation.

CYSTIC DISEASES OF THE KIDNEY

Overview

Cystic diseases of the kidney include a spectrum of diseases comprising hereditary, developmental and acquired disorders. They can result if the ureteric bud or kidney tissue fails to develop. Some of these diseases can lead to chronic renal failure (CRF). Diagnosis is made by finding multiple cysts on ultrasound. A single simple cyst is not an uncommon finding and should be considered normal.

Cystic renal dysplasia

This is an area of undifferentiated mesenchyme or cartilage within the parenchyma. It can be unilateral

Fig. 4.1 A horseshoe kidney.

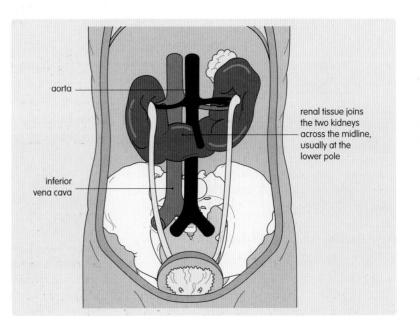

aorta

inferior vena cava

renal tissue joins the two kidneys across the midline, usually at the lower pole

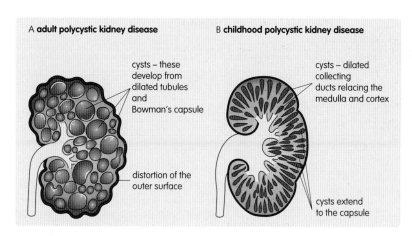

Fig. 4.2 Polycystic (A) adult and (B) childhood kidney disease.

(better prognosis) or bilateral, and is often associated with obstructive abnormalities in the ureter and lower urinary tract. Presentation is in childhood as an abdominal mass, and it is treated with surgical excision.

Polycystic kidney disease

Adult – autosomal dominant

Incidence and presenting features
This type of polycystic kidney disease accounts for 8–10% of CRF. Inheritance is autosomal dominant, and this is the most common inherited nephropathy. Three polycystic kidney disease (PKD) genes have been identified:

- *PKD 1*: on chromosome 16 (accounts for 85% of cases)
- *PKD 2*: on chromosome 4 (accounts for 10% of cases)
- *PKD 3*: accounts for a minority of cases and has yet to be mapped.

These mutations are thought to alter tubular epithelium growth and differentiation. Presentation is at 30–40 years of age with complications of hypertension, acute loin pain and/or haematuria, or bilateral large palpable kidneys. End-stage renal failure can develop, usually in the fifth or sixth decade of life. The disease is diagnosed increasingly earlier in life, as relatives of affected individuals are screened with abdominal ultrasound.

Pathology
Cysts develop anywhere in the kidney when dilatations in the nephron (Fig. 4.2A) compress the surrounding parenchyma and impair renal function. Sites for cyst formation are:

- Both kidneys
- Liver (lined by biliary epithelium) in 30–40% of cases
- Pancreas, lungs, ovaries, spleen and other organs.

Complications include uraemia, hypertension and berry aneurysms (found in 10–20% of cases). These develop as a result of congenital weakness in the arteries and increased blood pressure; they can lead to subarachnoid or cerebral haemorrhage.

Macroscopically, the kidneys are large with clear yellow fluid-filled cysts replacing the parenchyma. Haemorrhage into the cysts can occur. Microscopically, the cysts are lined by cuboidal epithelium.

Diagnosis
Large, irregular kidneys, and possibly hepatomegaly, are found on physical examination.

Diagnosis is made by:

- Ultrasound or computed tomography (CT): this shows bilateral enlarged kidneys with multiple cysts
- Genetic testing in families known to carry the PKD gene.

Prognosis
Morbidity and mortality are often the result of hypertension, for example myocardial infarction and cerebrovascular disease. The condition also leads to progressive chronic kidney disease (CKD). Rarely, complications are produced by the extrarenal cysts.

Treatment

This involves controlling blood pressure. Dialysis and renal transplant are needed if end-stage renal failure develops.

Child – autosomal recessive

Incidence and presenting features

This rare condition presents with enlarged kidneys or stillbirth. Both sexes are affected equally and more than one gene might be involved.

Pathology

Macroscopically, large kidneys with a radial pattern of fusiform-like cysts (sunburst pattern) are seen. Both kidneys are enlarged by multiple dilated collecting ducts which form the cysts. These replace the medulla and cortex and extend into the capsule (see Fig. 4.2B). The liver is almost always affected, with cysts, bile duct cell proliferation, fibrosis interfering with liver function and eventual portal hypertension.

Diagnosis, prognosis and treatment

Diagnosis is based on the presence of a palpable mass and ultrasound findings. Treatment involves managing the renal failure, hypertension and respiratory problems.

The prognosis is poor and death usually occurs due to renal or respiratory failure within the first few weeks of life, unless renal replacement therapy is given. Some children can survive for several years with independent renal function and develop portal hypertension and hepatic fibrosis.

Cystic diseases of the renal medulla

Nephronophthisis

Incidence and presenting features

This is an autosomal recessive condition that presents by the age of 25. Clinical features are polydipsia, polyuria, growth retardation and eventual renal failure. The disorder can coexist with retinal degeneration, optic atrophy, retinitis pigmentosa (giving tunnel vision), Laurence–Moon–Biedl syndrome or congenital hepatic fibrosis.

Pathology

Macroscopically, the kidneys appear small and fibrosed. Microscopically, there is interstitial inflammation and tubular atrophy. Later, multiple small medullary cysts develop.

Diagnosis, prognosis and treatment

Diagnosis is made from the family history and renal biopsy (this shows chronic tubulointerstitial nephritis). The disorder results in progressive renal failure, and treatment involves dialysis and renal transplantation.

Medullary sponge kidney

Incidence and presenting features

This is uncommon (1 in 20 000). It usually presents at 30–40 years of age with symptoms of urinary tract infection (UTI), stone formation or haematuria.

Pathology

Dilated collecting ducts in the medulla result in multiple cyst formation, mainly in the papillae (Fig. 4.3). Small calculi can develop within the cysts. One, part of one, or both kidneys can be affected. Macroscopically, some cysts are seen extending into the medulla from the involved calyces. In severe cases, the medulla looks spongy.

Diagnosis, prognosis and treatment

Diagnosis is by intravenous urography (IVU). The prognosis is good, with renal function remaining intact. A partial nephrectomy might be required.

Acquired cystic disease (dialysis associated)

Acquired cystic disease occurs in patients with CKD who have received dialysis for some time. The damaged kidneys develop many small cysts throughout the cortex and medulla, caused by obstruction of the tubules by interstitial fibrosis. The cysts have an atypical hyperplastic epithelial lining that can undergo malignant change.

Simple cysts

These are very common, with incidence increasing with age. They vary in size (usually 2–5 cm in diameter) and number, and contain clear fluid. Microscopically, they have a cuboidal epithelial lining and a thin capsule. Renal function is not affected but pain might be felt if there is haemorrhage into the cyst. The cysts can be differentiated from tumours by ultrasound (solid mass versus cystic mass).

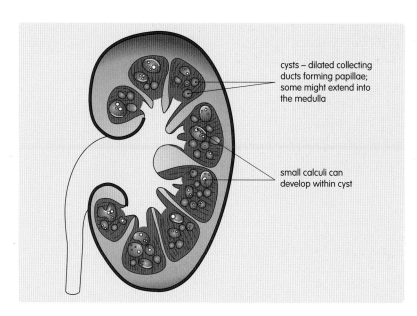

Fig. 4.3 Medullary sponge kidney.

cysts – dilated collecting ducts forming papillae; some might extend into the medulla

small calculi can develop within cyst

DISEASES OF THE GLOMERULUS

Overview

Glomerular disease (usually called glomerulonephritis (GN)) can be classified as:

- Hereditary (e.g. Alport's and Fabry's syndromes).
- Primary (most common): disease process originates from the glomerulus.
- Secondary to systemic diseases: e.g. diabetes mellitus, systemic lupus erythematosus (SLE), bacterial endocarditis.

> Polycystic kidney disease results in cysts developing anywhere in the kidney, causing dilatations in the nephron, and compression of the parenchyma, thus impairing renal function.

Hereditary glomerular disease

Alport's syndrome

This is usually X-linked, affecting mainly males (females are usually asymptomatic carriers). Autosomal dominant and autosomal recessive patterns of inheritance have also been described. An abnormality of basement membrane collagen IV is found in all patients, and they lack the Goodpasture's antigen.

Presentation is with glomerulonephritis and haematuria, ocular abnormalities and sensorineural deafness. Ocular lesions include lens dislocation, cataract and conical cornea. It is also associated with platelet dysfunction and hyperproteinaemia.

A few patients develop end-stage renal failure in childhood and adolescence. Females might have microscopic haematuria, but rarely develop end-stage renal failure. Treatment involves dialysis and/or transplantation.

Fabry's syndrome

This is a rare X-linked disorder, with a glycolipid metabolism defect due to the deficiency of galactosidase A. As a result, ceramide trihexoside (a glycosphingolipid) accumulates and is deposited in the kidneys, skin and vascular system. This disorder is associated with cardiac problems such as angina and cardiac failure – consequently, most patients die in the fifth decade of life.

Clinical manifestations of glomerular disease

Glomerular disease usually presents in one of the following five ways (Fig. 4.4):

1. Asymptomatic haematuria and proteinuria
2. Acute nephritic syndrome
3. Rapidly progressive glomerular disease
4. Nephrotic syndrome
5. CRF.

Fig. 4.4 Summary of types of glomerular disease and their clinical presentation

Clinical presentation	Primary glomerular cause	Secondary cause
asymptomatic haematuria	mesangial IgA glomerulonephritis (GN) other GN exercise-induced haemoglobinuria	Henoch–Schönlein purpura (HSP) systemic lupus erythematosus (SLE) bacterial endocarditis
asymptomatic proteinuria	mesangial capillary GN any other GN focal segmental glomerulosclerosis shunt nephritis any cause of renal scarring	HSP SLE bacterial endocarditis polyarteritis nodosa severe long-standing hypertension pregnancy
acute nephritic syndrome	post-streptococcal GN non-streptococcal GN rapidly progressive GN focal proliferative GN mesangial IgA GN	SLE microscopic polyangiitis Wegener's granulomatosis
nephrotic syndrome	minimal change disease membranous glomerulonephropathy membranoproliferative GN focal segmental glomerulosclerosis shunt nephritis (rare)	HSP SLE tumour amyloid diabetes mellitus drugs (e.g. penicillamine, gold) bacterial endocarditis congenital nephrotic syndrome
chronic renal failure glomerulosclerosis	this develops as a long-term consequence of any of above diseases	

Four structures within the glomerulus are prone to damage:

- Capillary endothelial cell lining
- Glomerular basement membrane
- Mesangium supporting the capillaries
- Podocytes on the outer surface of the capillary

When damage occurs to the glomerulus, it often results in painless haematuria, and can be continuous or intermittent.

Asymptomatic haematuria

Haematuria due to glomerular disease is often painless and can be continuous or intermittent. Primary and secondary causes are summarized in Figure 4.4. It should be noted that heavy exercise can result in haemoglobinuria (not haematuria).

Asymptomatic proteinuria

This is characterized by proteinuria (usually 0.3–3 g protein daily) with no other symptoms. Possible causes are summarized in Figure 4.4.

Acute nephritic syndrome

The symptoms and signs are:

- Oliguria/anuria
- Hypertension
- Fluid retention – seen as facial oedema
- Haematuria – microscopic or macroscopic
- Uraemia
- Proteinuria.

Patients might also complain of loin pain, headache and general malaise. Primary and secondary causes of acute nephritic syndrome are summarized in Figure 4.4.

Rapidly progressive GN

Rapidly progressive GN, or crescentic GN, occurs when there is severe glomerular injury. It presents with haematuria, oliguria and hypertension, eventually causing renal failure.

Nephrotic syndrome

This is characterized by:

- Proteinuria (typically >3 g/24 h) – sufficient to cause:
- Hypoalbuminaemia (serum albumin typically <25 g/L) – sufficient to cause:
- Oedema and secondary hypercholesterolaemia.

There is increased permeability of the glomerular filter to albumin as a result of glomerular basement membrane damage and increase in pore size. The capillary wall becomes permeable to proteins of higher molecular weight as the severity of injury increases. Heavy proteinuria leads to low plasma albumin and therefore tissue oedema.

In an adult a loss of more than 3–5 g of albumin per day can cause hypoalbuminaemia, but some patients can have nephrotic-range proteinuria without being overtly nephrotic, because the rate of albumin synthesis compensates for the albumin loss. A limited amount of filtered protein can be reabsorbed by endocytosis, but if this is exceeded, protein is lost in the urine. The albumin content within the capillary helps maintain the colloid osmotic pressure. If this decreases, less fluid moves back into the capillaries, causing oedema in the peripheral tissues. The decreased circulating volume stimulates the renin–angiotensin–aldosterone system, leading to further sodium and water retention, and further oedema.

Treatment

Management includes:

- Blood pressure control
- Reduction of proteinuria, using angiotensin-converting enzyme (ACE) inhibitors
- Control of hyperlipidaemia
- Anticoagulation if hypercoagulable (risk of thrombosis increases as albumin decreases)
- Treatment of underlying causes when possible, e.g. in minimal change disease high-dose corticosteroid therapy will eliminate proteinuria in up to 90% of cases.

Complications of nephrotic syndrome include:

- Hypercoagulable state: increases risk of deep vein thrombosis, pulmonary embolus and renal vein thrombosis.
- Hyperlipidaemia: increases risk of vascular disease and ischaemic heart disease.
- Immunosuppression: increases risk of infection.

Primary and secondary causes are summarized in Figure 4.4.

Chronic renal failure

CRF results from any disease causing progressive nephron loss. The kidney shrinks, with cortical thinning. Most of the glomeruli are replaced by hyaline balls, and there is almost complete tubular atrophy. This is often asymptomatic in the early stages. Later, symptoms develop as waste products accumulate and erythropoietin or vitamin D production is reduced. Symptoms include:

- Uraemia
- Hypertension
- Salt and water retention causing oedema
- Anaemia
- Nausea, vomiting, diarrhoea
- Gastrointestinal bleeding
- Itching
- Polyuria and nocturia
- Lethargy
- Paraesthesiae (due to polyneuropathy)
- Mental slowing and clouding of consciousness (terminal stage).

In extreme cases, oliguria results. Dialysis or renal transplantation are effective treatments.

The mechanisms of glomerular injury

Circulating immune complex nephritis

This is the most common mechanism of immune-mediated damage. Immune complexes form outside the kidney and become trapped in the glomerulus after travelling to the kidney via the renal circulation (Fig. 4.5B). The antigen can be:

- Exogenous: bacteria (e.g. group A streptococci such as *Treponema pallidum*), surface antigen of hepatitis B, hepatitis C virus antigen, tumour antigens, viruses.
- Endogenous: DNA in SLE.

When trapped in the glomerulus, the immune complexes activate the classical complement pathway, causing acute inflammation of the glomerulus. Immunofluorescence microscopy demonstrates immunoglobulin deposits along the basement membrane and/or in the mesangium. These increase vascular permeability.

In situ immune complex deposition

Antigen–antibody immune complexes form within the kidney when antibodies react with intrinsic or planted antigens within the glomerulus (Fig. 4.5A).

Antiglomerular basement membrane (anti-GBM) disease is an example of reaction to intrinsic antigens. Antibodies are formed against an antigen in the GBM, to form a complex which stimulates the complement cascade. This damages the glomerulus and leads to rapidly progressing renal failure. The anti-GBM antibodies also attack the basement membrane of the alveoli in the lungs. The triad of anti-GBM antibodies, GN and pulmonary haemorrhage is known as Goodpasture's syndrome.

Reaction to planted antigens occurs when circulating antigens are deposited within the glomerulus. They can be:

- Exogenous: e.g. bacteria such as group A β-haemolytic streptococci, which cause post-streptococcal GN. Other antigens include bacterial products (endostreptosin), aggregated IgG, viruses, parasites and drugs.
- Endogenous: e.g. anti-DNA antibodies react with circulating DNA (as seen in SLE).

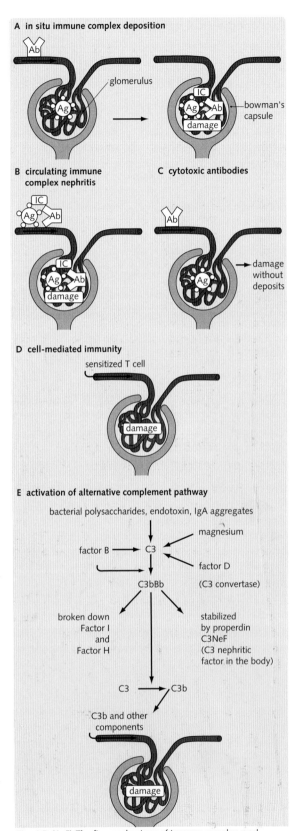

Fig. 4.5 (A–E) The five mechanisms of immune complex renal disease. Ab, antibody; Ag, antigen; IC, immune complex.

Cell-mediated immunity

Sensitized T cells from cell-mediated immune reactions play a role in the progression of acute GN to chronic GN (Fig. 4.5D). Glomerular damage is thought to be mediated by macrophages and T lymphocytes.

Activation of alternative complement pathway

Bacterial polysaccharides, endotoxins, and IgA aggregates can stimulate the alternative complement pathway – the products of which deposit in the glomeruli, impairing glomerular function (Fig. 4.5E). This occurs in membranoproliferative GN.

Cytotoxic antibodies

Antibodies to glomerular cell antigens cause damage without the formation and deposition of immune complexes (Fig. 4.5C). This is uncommon. An example would be antibody fixing to mesangial cells, resulting in complement-mediated mesangiolysis and mesangial cell proliferation.

Acute glomerulonephritis

Post-streptococcal glomerulonephritis

This presents 1–3 weeks following a group A β-haemolytic streptococcal infection of the tonsils, pharynx or skin. Clinical features include proteinuria, haematuria and a low glomerular filtration rate (GFR) (this causes fluid retention, oligaemia and hypertension). All the glomeruli are involved thus resulting in a diffuse proliferative GN – 'proliferative' because there is an increase in the cellularity in the glomerulus. Treatment is usually conservative, with antibiotics to treat any remaining infection. The prognosis is excellent in children but only 60% of adults recover completely; the rest develop hypertension or renal impairment.

Non-streptococcal glomerulonephritis

Non-streptococcal GN follows a similar process to that for post-streptococcal GN except that the causative organism is not a streptococcus. It can be triggered by:

- Other bacteria (i.e. staphylococci and pneumococci).

- Parasites (*Toxoplasma gondii, Plasmodium*).
- Viruses.

Glomerular disease is classified as:

- Focal – affects only some glomeruli
- Diffuse – affects all the glomeruli
- Segmental – affects only part of the glomerulus
- Global – affects the entire glomerulus.

Rapidly progressive (crescentic) glomerulonephritis

This results in severe glomerular injury. Histologically, glomerular injury results in leakage of fibrin, which stimulates epithelial cells and macrophages within Bowman's capsule to proliferate and form crescent-shaped masses, reducing glomerular blood supply. It can be seen as part of systemic illnesses such as SLE, Wegener's granulomatosis and microscopic polyangiitis. As the name suggests, the disease progresses rapidly and there is a loss of renal function within days to weeks. Prompt diagnosis and treatment is therefore required to prevent hypertension, kidney scarring and renal failure. Treatment consists of high-dose steroids, immunosuppressants and plasma exchange.

Minimal change disease

This is the most common cause of nephrotic syndrome in children under the age of 6 years, and more commonly affects males. No significant renal changes are seen under the light microscope (hence the name). Electron microscopy shows podocyte fusion, i.e. foot process effacement. The cause is unknown, but potential mechanisms include a post-allergic reaction, circulating immune complexes, or altered T-cell immunity. Treatment involves corticosteroid therapy and ciclosporin or cyclophosphamide (if resistant). The prognosis is good in children and variable in adults, but usually good. Occasionally, this disorder causes end-stage renal failure.

Membranous glomerulonephropathy

This is a chronic disease characterized by:

- Subepithelial deposition of immune complexes.
- Basement membrane thickening.

It accounts for 40% of adult nephrotic syndrome and is more common in males. Causes are idiopathic (85%), primary or secondary. Secondary causes include:

- Infections: syphilis, malaria, hepatitis B.
- Tumours: melanoma, carcinoma of the bronchus, lymphoma.
- Drugs: penicillamine, heroin, mercury, gold.
- Systemic illnesses: SLE.

Histological examination reveals widespread glomerular basement thickening caused by immunoglobulin deposition. Over time, the abnormal excess mesangial matrix causes hyalinization of the glomerulus and death of individual nephrons. Drug treatment involves corticosteroids, cyclophosphamide, ciclosporin and chlorambucil. Prognosis depends on the cause; 30% of idiopathic cases develop CRF and require dialysis or transplantation. In secondary membranous glomerulonephropathy, treatment of underlying disease causes disease remission. Complications of membranous glomerulopathy are the same as those for nephrotic syndrome (see p. 71).

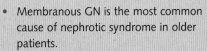
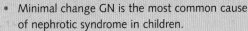

- Membranous GN is the most common cause of nephrotic syndrome in older patients.
- Minimal change GN is the most common cause of nephrotic syndrome in children.

Membranoproliferative glomerulonephropathy

This is common in children and young adults, and more common in females than males. It is characterized histologically by diffuse global basement membrane thickening and mesangial proliferation. It is usually primary, but can be secondary to disorders such as SLE and malaria. Primary membranoproliferative GN is classified as:

- Type I (more common): immune complexes deposit in the subendothelium, causing inflammation and capillary thickening. This occurs in infections, tumours, drug reactions, genetic disorders, connective tissue disorders (e.g. SLE) and complement deficiencies.

- Type II: caused by activation of the alternative complement pathway (dense deposit disease) following an infection. Histological examination reveals thickened capillaries caused by C3 deposition. It is associated with partial lipodystrophy.

Clinically, types I and II are indistinguishable, presenting with asymptomatic haematuria or combined nephrotic/nephritic syndrome. Prognosis is poor – the disease progresses to end-stage renal failure. Treatment involves dialysis and renal transplantation. Recurrence occurs following transplant, particularly in type II disease.

Focal segmental glomerulosclerosis

This accounts for 10% of childhood and up to 30% of cases of adult nephrotic syndrome. It is more common in males and its causes are:

- Altered cellular immunity
- Intravenous heroin use
- Acquired immune deficiency syndrome
- Reaction to chronic proteinuria
- Idiopathic.

Histological examination reveals focal collapse and sclerosis, with hyaline deposits in glomerular segments. Presentation is with proteinuria or nephrotic syndrome, later developing haematuria and hypertension. Most develop CRF within 10 years. Treatment of the idiopathic form involves steroids, cyclophosphamide, ciclosporin, dialysis and renal transplantation. Recurrence can be seen after a renal transplant.

Focal proliferative glomerulonephritis

Focal proliferative GN results in inflammation of some parts of some glomeruli. Its presentation is less acute. It might affect only the kidney (IgA nephropathy, see below) or be secondary to systemic illnesses such as Henoch–Schönlein purpura (HSP), Goodpasture's syndrome, subacute bacterial endocarditis, vasculitis and other connective tissue diseases (e.g. SLE). Treatment with immunosuppression can be effective. The prognosis is variable. Necrotizing GN is also often seen in malignant hypertension.

IgA nephropathy (Berger's disease)

This is the most common primary glomerular disease worldwide, causing recurrent haematuria. There is some association with geographical location (more common in France, Australia and Singapore) and human leucocyte antigen (HLA) DR4. It typically affects young men after an upper respiratory tract infection. Presentation is with microscopic haematuria and proteinuria and renal impairment. There is hypertension and plasma IgA levels are raised. Histologically, IgA and C3 deposits are seen in the mesangium of all the glomeruli, with some mesangial proliferation (this is similar to the histological picture seen in HSP). Eventually, there is sclerosis of the damaged segment. There is no effective treatment. Patients with late onset, proteinuria, increased blood pressure and increased creatinine at presentation have a worse prognosis – up to 20% of patients develop end-stage renal failure.

Chronic glomerulonephritis

There is diffuse global glomerular destruction and hyalinization associated with CRF. The kidneys are small with granular scarring. Chronic GN is the end-stage result of several types of GN; in particular, rapidly progressive GN, focal glomerulosclerosis, membranoproliferative GN and IgA nephropathy, although when advanced it is usually not possible to define the initial insult. Histological examination reveals:

- Glomeruli hyalinization
- Tubular atrophy
- Interstitial fibrosis.

Unlike chronic pyelonephritis, the pelvicalyceal system is unaffected in chronic GN. Instead, the kidneys are small, with diffuse global glomerular destruction associated with CRF.

GLOMERULAR LESIONS IN SYSTEMIC DISEASE

Systemic disorders can cause glomerular disease. They are usually:

- Immune complex mediated (e.g. SLE, HSP, bacterial endocarditis)

- Vascular (e.g. microscopic polyangiitis, Wegener's granulomatosis)
- Metabolic (e.g. diabetes mellitus, amyloidosis)
- Drug treatment (e.g. penicillamine, gold, captopril, phenytoin)
- Infections (e.g. hepatitis B, leprosy, syphilis, malaria).

Systemic lupus erythematosus

SLE is an autoimmune vasculitis characterized by antinuclear antibodies and widespread immune-complex-mediated inflammation. It is more common in females, Asians and if an individual is HLA B8, DR2 or DR3 positive. It is a relapsing and remitting condition, usually diagnosed between 30 and 40 years of age. It affects many systems and organs in the body; for example, the joints, skin, heart, lungs and the kidneys (75% of cases). The renal lesions are the most important clinically and affect prognosis. Glomerular changes vary from minimal involvement to diffuse proliferative disease with:

- Immune complex deposition in glomerulus (frequently all classes of immunoglobulin and complement)
- Basement membrane thickening
- Endothelial proliferation.

This results in focal or diffuse proliferative GN, or membranous glomerulopathy. Patients present with proteinuria, oedema and hypertension. There may be extrarenal systemic symptoms. Patients may develop CRF, but the prognosis is improved with immunosuppressive treatment (steroids, azathioprine or cyclophosphamide).

Henoch–Schönlein purpura

HSP is seen predominantly in children, affecting males more than females. It is an immune-mediated systemic vasculitis that affects many parts of the body including:

- Skin: a purpuric rash is seen over on the extensor surface of the legs, arms and buttocks.
- Joints: resulting in pain.
- Intestine: resulting in abdominal pain, vomiting, bleeding.
- Kidney: resulting in GN (a third of patients develop glomerular lesions histologically identical to IgA nephropathy).

Fig. 4.6 Summary of the natural history of diabetes. 'Asterisk' (*) indicates functional changes in kidney size (increased) and short-term glomerular filtration rate (increased). ESRD, end-stage renal disease.

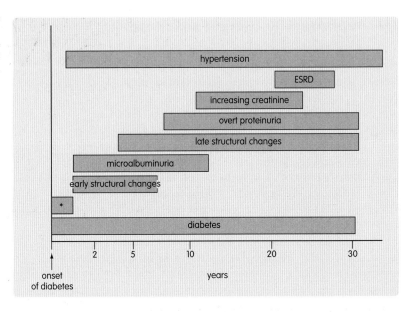

HSP can follow an upper respiratory tract infection. It has an excellent prognosis in children.

Bacterial endocarditis

Glomerular disease in bacterial endocarditis is caused by:

- Immune complex deposits in the glomerulus
- Embolism-mediated infarction – emboli break away from the heart valves.

The main histological diagnoses are focal, segmental and diffuse proliferative GN. Presentation is with microscopic haematuria, fluid retention and renal impairment. Renal lesions resolve on antibiotic therapy.

Diabetic glomerulosclerosis

Diabetes mellitus affects several organs including the kidneys, which are the most commonly and severely damaged organs in diabetes. Diabetic nephropathy is the most common cause of requiring dialysis treatment in developed countries. Renal manifestations include nodular glomerulosclerosis (described later) and arteriosclerosis, including benign nephrosclerosis with hypertension (Figure 4.6 presents a summary of the natural history of diabetes). Histological features can include:

- Thickening of the capillary basement membrane
- Increase in the matrix of the mesangium

- A diffuse or nodular pattern of glomerulosclerosis (also known as Kimmelstiel–Wilson syndrome)
- Arterial hyalinosis of both the afferent and efferent arterioles – this predisposes to vessel occlusion.

The arteries can also be affected (especially in type II diabetes) and severe atheroma in the renal artery leads to renal ischaemia and hypertension. Papillary necrosis is a recognized complication, especially in the presence of infection. Diabetic nephropathy presents with microalbuminuria, which increases progressively to nephrotic range proteinuria (i.e. >3 g/24 h). Consequently, GFR gradually declines, leading to CRF, which can be seen in 30% of cases of insulin-dependent type 1 diabetes mellitus. It is also associated with diabetic complications elsewhere (e.g. retinopathy in the eyes). Chronic renal damage as a result of diabetes is associated and accelerated by hypertension.

Treatment includes ACE inhibitors to reduce proteinuria (these are discussed later), strict blood pressure and glycaemic control, and dialysis for end-stage renal failure.

Amyloidosis

This disorder involves deposition of amyloid (an extracellular fibrillar protein) in the glomeruli, usually within the mesangium and subendothelium, and sometimes in the subepithelial space. Deposits can also be found in the walls of the blood vessels and in the interstitium. Clinically, this results in heavy proteinuria or the nephrotic syndrome, eventually leading to CRF (due to ischaemia and glomerulosclerosis). Dialysis or transplant is required to prevent death from uraemia.

Goodpasture's syndrome

In Goodpasture's syndrome, autoantibodies to type IV collagen in the glomerular basement membrane develop, causing inflammation. Presentation is with a rapidly progressive 'crescentic' GN and acute renal failure (ARF) and lung haemorrhage. Prognosis is poor without treatment, which involves:

- Plasma exchange (to remove the antibodies)
- Corticosteroids (to reduce inflammation).

Microscopic polyarteritis nodosa (also known as microscopic polyangiitis)

This is a necrotizing vasculitis affecting the small arteries of the body; it is more common in males. Initially, there is a focal, segmental or necrotizing GN followed by rapidly progressive GN. Histological examination reveals extensive necrosis, fibrin deposition and epithelial crescents. Microscopic polyarteritis nodosa (PAN) is associated with circulating antineutrophil cytoplasmic antibodies (ANCA), which complex with a perinuclear antigen (myeloperoxidase) in fixed neutrophils (pANCA).

Wegener's granulomatosis

This is a rare necrotizing vasculitis affecting the nose, upper respiratory tract and kidneys. It typically presents between 40 and 50 years of age. The glomerular disease is similar to that in microscopic PAN, with granuloma formation. Presentation is with asymptomatic haematuria or nephritic syndrome (focal segmental GN) or rapidly progressive GN. It is associated with ANCA, which characteristically recognizes a cytoplasmic antigen (proteinase 3) in fixed neutrophils (cANCA).

Hereditary nephritis

This is a spectrum of conditions, usually inherited, which present as GN with haematuria, often progressing to renal failure (e.g. Alport's syndrome, see p. 69).

DISEASES OF THE TUBULES AND INTERSTITIUM

Overview

The tubules and interstitium are affected by several diseases. Typically, tubules become obstructed (this reduces glomerular filtration) or their transport functions become impaired (reduces water and solute reabsorption). Damage can be acute or chronic.

Acute tubular necrosis

Acute tubular necrosis (ATN) is the result of acute tubular cell damage by ischaemia or toxins. It can be oliguric (<400 mL/day urine) or non-oliguric. Hyperkalaemia can develop as a result of K^+ retention and this can trigger cardiac arrhythmias, which can be life-threatening. Uraemia develops because there is a significant fall in GFR – this could be due to haemodynamic changes and intratubular obstruction. Recovery is accompanied by a diuretic phase that occurs because of failure to concentrate urine (this can cause hypokalaemia).

ATN is a cause of ARF. Mortality is up to 50% but full recovery is possible with prompt treatment – fluid and electrolyte therapy and dialysis if necessary.

Ischaemic acute tubular necrosis

This is caused by hypotension and hypovolaemic shock following trauma, infections, burns or haemorrhage. There is a rapid fall in blood pressure, which causes hypoperfusion of the peritubular capillaries with consequent tubular necrosis along the entire length of the nephron. The kidneys appear pale and swollen. Histological examination reveals:

- Infiltration of inflammatory cells and the tubular cells
- Flattened and vacuolated tubular cells
- Interstitial oedema
- Cellular debris and protein casts in the distal tubule and the collecting ducts
- Myoglobin in the casts in crush injuries.

Non-steroidal anti-inflammatory drugs (NSAIDs) can increase the risk of ATN following other renal insults by preventing the synthesis of prostaglandins (PGs). PGs are vasodilators, which protect the kidney from ischaemic injury by dilating blood vessels and increasing blood flow.

Toxic acute tubular necrosis

This disorder is caused by agents with specific nephrotoxic activity causing damage to the epithelial cells. Such substances include:

- Organic solvents: carbon tetrachloride (CCl_4) in dry-cleaning fluid
- Heavy metals (gold, mercury, lead and arsenic)
- Antibiotics (gentamicin)
- Pesticides.

These substances cause the cells to come away from the basement membrane and consequently collect in and obstruct the tubular lumen. The effect is limited because there is regeneration of the epithelial cells in 10–20 days, which permits clinical recovery and is confirmed by the presence of mitotic figures on biopsy. Damage by nephrotoxic substances is limited to the proximal tubules. The kidneys appear swollen and red.

Tubulointerstitial nephritis

Urinary tract infection

Incidence and risk factors

Urinary tract infections (UTIs) are very common. They can involve the bladder (cystitis) or the kidneys (pyelonephritis) or both. UTIs are more common in boys in infancy because of congenital abnormalities; this reverses at puberty, with more females being affected thereafter because of urethral trauma and pregnancy. Women are particularly at risk of lower UTIs because they have a short urethra, but further investigation is required if infections are recurrent. Any UTI in children and men should be investigated to exclude an underlying renal tract abnormality. UTIs rarely progress to renal damage in adults if the renal tract is normal. Treatment involves a high fluid intake, regular bladder emptying and prophylactic antibiotics. After the age of 40, UTI is again more common in men because of prostatic disease, causing bladder outflow obstruction. Risk factors for UTIs include:

- Long-term catheterization
- Diabetes mellitus
- Lower urinary tract obstruction (congenital abnormalities or calculi)
- Pregnancy
- Tumours
- Immunosuppression
- VUR.

Fig. 4.7 Incidence of community- and hospital-acquired urinary tract infections (UTIs) caused by bacteria

Organism	Community (%)	Hospital (%)
Escherichia coli	80–90	45–55
Proteus	5–10	10–12
Klebsiella	1–2	15–20
Enterobacter	–	2–5
Pseudomonas	–	10–15
Acinetobacter	–	<1
coagulase-negative *Staphylococcus*	1–2	1–2
Staphylococcus aureus	–	<1
Enterococcus	<1	10–12

Presentation

UTIs present silently (asymptomatic bacteriuria) or with dysuria (pain on passing urine), frequency and urgency of micturition. Involvement of the kidneys causes loin pain and fever.

Diagnosis

A diagnosis of UTI requires over 10^5 organisms/mL from a midstream urine specimen on culture. In the majority of UTIs the infecting organism comes from the patient's own faecal flora (Fig. 4.7).

Pyelonephritis

This is a bacterial infection of the kidney and results in inflammation and damage to the renal calyces, parenchyma and pelvis. It can be acute or chronic.

Acute pyelonephritis

This occurs because of infection in the kidney and is spread via two routes:

1. Ascending infection: bacteria from the gut enter the kidney from the lower urinary tract if there is an incompetent vesicoureteric valve. This permits vesicoureteric reflux (VUR) and results in ascending transmission of infection.
2. Haematogenous spread: seen in patients with septicaemia or infective endocarditis. The pathogens include fungi, bacteria (staphylococci

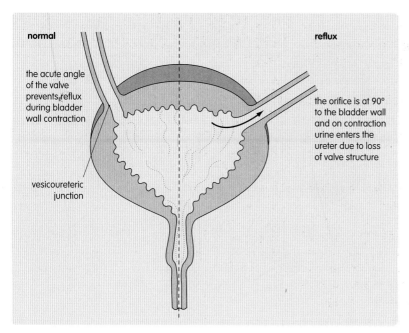

Fig. 4.8 Normal and refluxing (abnormal) junction.

normal

the acute angle of the valve prevents reflux during bladder wall contraction

vesicoureteric junction

reflux

the orifice is at 90° to the bladder wall and on contraction urine enters the ureter due to loss of valve structure

and *Escherichia coli*) and viruses. The kidney is often affected in septicaemic diseases because of its large blood supply.

The predisposing factors of acute pyelonephritis are:

- Urinary tract obstruction (congenital and acquired)
- VUR
- Instrumentation of the urinary tract
- Sexual intercourse
- Diabetes mellitus
- Immunosuppression (human immunodeficiency virus infection, lymphoma and transplants).

Patients present with general malaise, fever, loin pain, tenderness and often rigors with or without symptoms of lower UTI. Infection spreads into the renal pelvis and papillae and causes abscess formation throughout the cortex and medulla.

With retrograde ureteric spread the kidney characteristically contains areas of wedge-shaped suppuration especially at the upper and lower poles. In septicaemia there is haematogenous seeding within the kidney and minute abscesses are distributed randomly in the cortex. On histological examination there is:

- Polymorphic infiltration of the tubules
- Interstitial oedema
- Focal inflammation.

Uncomplicated cases resolve with antibiotic treatment and high fluid intake. The important complications of acute pyelonephritis are:

- Renal papillary necrosis
- Perinephric abscesses
- Pyonephrosis (obstruction of the pelvicalyceal system)
- Chronic pyelonephritis
- Fibrosis and scarring.

Chronic pyelonephritis

This condition is characterized by long-standing parenchymal scarring, which develops from tubulointerstitial inflammation. It is the end-result of various pathological processes. There are two main types:

1. Obstructive: chronic obstruction (stones, tumours or congenital abnormalities) prevents pelvicalyceal drainage and increases the risk of renal infection. Chronic pyelonephritis develops because of recurrent infection.
2. Reflux nephropathy: this is the most common cause of chronic pyelonephritis. It is associated with VUR, which is congenital. The organisms enter the ascending portion of the ureter with refluxed urine as the valvular orifice is held open on contraction of the bladder during micturition. Reflux results from the abnormal angle at which the ureter enters the bladder wall (Fig. 4.8).

Fig. 4.9 Differences between (A) acute and (B) chronic pyelonephritis.

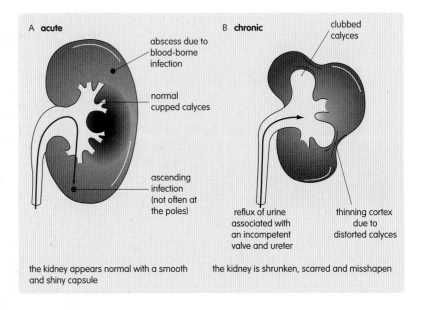

A **acute**

abscess due to blood-borne infection

normal cupped calyces

ascending infection (not often at the poles)

the kidney appears normal with a smooth and shiny capsule

B **chronic**

clubbed calyces

reflux of urine associated with an incompetent valve and ureter

thinning cortex due to distorted calyces

the kidney is shrunken, scarred and misshapen

The disease process usually begins in childhood and has a silent, insidious onset. Reflux of urine into the renal pelvis occurs during micturition and this increases the pressure in the major calyces. The high intrapelvic pressure forces urine into the collecting ducts with intraparenchymal reflux further distorting the internal structure. This is most predominant at the poles of the kidney and results in deep irregular scars on the cortical surface. The tubulointerstitial inflammation heals with the formation of cortico-medullary scars that overlie the deformed and dilated calyces, which are characteristic of chronic pyelonephritis (Fig. 4.9).

On histological examination there is interstitial fibrosis and dilated tubules containing eosinophilic casts; 10–20% of patients requiring dialysis have chronic pyelonephritis.

Ultrasonography is used to diagnose chronic pyelonephritis and may show distortion of the calyceal system and contraction of the kidney because of cortical scarring. Intravenous pyelography may be more sensitive but requires exposure to X-rays which should be avoided, especially in children.

Toxin- and drug-induced tubulointerstitial nephritis

Heavy metals (mercury, gold, lead) and drugs (ampicillin, rifampicin, NSAIDs) can cause T-cell-mediated inflammation in the interstitium. This reaction usually occurs 2–40 days after exposure to the toxin. Clinical features include fever, skin rash, haematuria, proteinuria and ARF. Withdrawal of the causative agent leads to recovery.

On histological examination there is interstitial oedema and tubular degeneration with eosinophil infiltration. In chronic analgesic abuse with phenacetin, and to a lesser extent aspirin, PG synthesis is inhibited, causing ischaemia (as described on p. 77 for ischaemic ATN). This causes papillary necrosis and a secondary tubulonephritis (analgesic nephropathy). It is associated with an increased risk of developing transitional cell carcinomas with chronic analgesic abuse.

Chronic analgesic misuse inhibits PG synthesis, causing ischaemia. The resultant papillary necrosis can be diagnosed in X-rays. It is seen in analgesic nephropathy, diabetes, sickle-cell disease and urinary tract obstruction.

Urate nephropathy

If there is an increased blood urate concentration, urate crystals are precipitated in the acidic environment of the collecting ducts, causing inflammatory obstruction and dilatation of the tubules. This eventually leads to fibrosis and atrophy. An increase in urate concentration can be caused by:

- Rapid cell turnover (e.g. in psoriasis or malignancy): in those patients with haematological or lymphatic malignancy who are receiving chemotherapy there is excess cell breakdown and release of nucleic acids, which results in acute urate nephropathy and ARF.

- Reduced uric acid clearance (e.g. in CRF): this is seen in patients with gout, in which there is a long-term deposition of urate in the kidney as a result of the constant high blood urate levels.

Urate nephropathy causes acute or chronic renal failure depending on the time-course of urate deposition:

- Patients with malignancy treated with chemotherapy are prone to ARF
- Patients with gout are prone to CRF.

Hypercalcaemia and nephrocalcinosis

A persistently high blood Ca^{2+} level causes Ca^{2+} deposition in the kidneys. The hypercalcaemia can be due to:

- Primary hyperparathyroidism
- Multiple myeloma
- Increased vitamin D activity
- Bone metastases.

Renal insufficiency occurs in these patients because of stones (nephrolithiasis) or focal calcification in the renal parenchyma (nephrocalcinosis).

In nephrocalcinosis the Ca^{2+} accumulates in the tubular cells and the basement membrane, resulting in interstitial fibrosis and inflammation. Hypercalcaemia also causes a renal concentrating defect, which leads to polyuria, nocturia and dehydration.

Multiple myeloma

Approximately 50% of patients with multiple myeloma develop renal insufficiency, which can cause ARF or CRF. Histological changes include:

- Bence Jones proteins (light chains) enter the urine and these are toxic to the tubular epithelial cells. They combine with Tamm–Horsfall protein to precipitate as casts in the tubules, causing inflammation and obstruction to the tubular cells
- Amyloid lambda (λ) or kappa (κ) light-chain fragments (paraproteins) are deposited in the renal blood vessels, glomeruli and tubules

- Urate deposition (discussed above)
- Hypercalcaemia (discussed above).

DISEASES OF THE RENAL BLOOD VESSELS

Benign nephrosclerosis

This is the term given to the changes in renal vasculature in response to long-standing essential (benign) hypertension. The changes consist of hyaline arteriolosclerosis, which is characterized by thickening (due to hyperplasia of smooth muscle) and hyalinization (protein deposition) of the arteriolar wall. This causes narrowing of the lumen of the interlobular arteries, which functionally impairs the smaller branches. The changes are more severe in patients with systemic diseases that affect the renal vessels (e.g. diabetes). The vascular wall lesions gradually reduce the blood supply to the kidney, which leads to ischaemic atrophy of the nephrons. This accounts for the small, contracted and granular appearance of the kidneys seen in advanced cases of untreated essential hypertension. Renal function may be well preserved initially, although proteinuria is sometimes detected.

Malignant nephrosclerosis

This is associated with accelerated hypertension. It occurs in 1–5% of patients with hypertension. There is a sudden accelerated rise in blood pressure with an increase in diastolic pressure to over 130 mmHg. In acute cases the kidney surface appears smooth and is covered in tiny petechial haemorrhages. There are fibrin deposits in the vessel wall, causing necrosis (fibrinoid necrosis), especially in the distal part of the interlobular arteries and the afferent arterioles.

Renal function is impaired because of the ischaemia that results from severe arterial damage. Patients have proteinuria and haematuria, which can occasionally be massive. Renal failure develops if untreated (in contrast to benign hypertension). Papilloedema is often present. The 5-year survival rate with treatment is 50%.

The trigger for the abrupt and rapid rise in blood pressure is unknown but might be associated with endothelial dysfunction. These patients also have increased plasma levels of renin, aldosterone and angiotensin.

Fig. 4.10 Comparison between fibromuscular dysplasia and atheromatous renal artery stenosis (RAS)

	Fibromuscular dysplasia	Atheromatous RAS
age (years)	<40	>55
sex prevalence	F > M	M > F
bruit heard	80%	40%
vascular disease	rare	common elsewhere
renal failure	rare	well recognized
prognosis	good	poor

Renal artery stenosis

Between 2% and 5% of hypertensive patients have hypertension secondary to renal artery stenosis (RAS) in one or both renal arteries. This is narrowing of the renal arteries caused by atheromatous plaques (70%) or fibromuscular dysplasia within the renal artery wall (Fig. 4.10). Poor renal perfusion is interpreted by the affected kidney as a fall in body fluid volume, which stimulates renin secretion. Ischaemia of the affected kidney leads to a small kidney.

Treatment options include:

- **Drugs to control the blood pressure and vascular risk factors**: If the blood pressure is left uncontrolled the contralateral kidney may become damaged by hypertension.
- **Angioplasty**: to dilate the stenotic region. This can be supplemented with stenting to decrease the risk of restenosis.
- **Bypass surgery**: of the narrowed vessels (now rarely undertaken).
- **Nephrectomy**.

The benefits of correcting RAS either in terms of controlling blood pressure or delaying progression of CKD have not been fully evaluated in atherosclerotic RAS.

Thrombotic microangiopathies

This is a group of diseases that are all characterized by necrosis and thickening of the renal vessel walls and thrombosis in the interlobular arterioles, afferent arterioles and glomeruli. All clinically present with the triad of:

- Haemolysis
- Thrombocytopenia
- ARF.

The main two microangiopathies are:

1. Haemolytic uraemic syndrome (HUS)
2. Thrombotic thrombocytopenic purpura (TTP).

Haemolytic uraemic syndrome

This is characterized by the triad of:

- Microangiopathic haemolytic anaemia
- Thrombocytopenia (decreased platelets)
- Renal failure (with normal clotting).

It is classified as:

- **Idiopathic**: this is more common in adults, and has a worse prognosis.
- **Secondary**: this can be associated with gastroenteritis (e.g. *Escherichia coli* 0157 toxin), drugs (oestrogen, ciclosporin, cytotoxic therapy) or malignancy. HUS can also be caused by accelerated hypertension or, more rarely, there might be a genetic cause.

Clinical features include sudden onset of oliguria with haematuria – occasionally with malaena or haematemesis (usually if gastroenteritis is the cause) – and jaundice. Hypertension is seen in 50% of patients.

Treatment involves early supportive therapy with dialysis for renal failure. Fresh frozen plasma or plasma exchange can be useful. Approximately 50% of patients later develop hypertension, and a few go on to develop CRF. Mortality ranges from 5% to 30%.

Thrombotic thrombocytopenic purpura

This is a rare and idiopathic condition that is more common in females (usually <40 years) than in males. The features are fever, neurological signs (central nervous system (CNS) involvement), haemolytic anaemia and thrombocytopenia. TTP has a similar disease process to HUS, but affects different sites. Renal involvement occurs in only 50% of cases, and presents with:

- Proteinuria
- Haematuria
- Renal insufficiency.

The majority of cases have a dominant CNS component, with thrombosis leading to ischaemia in the brain.

Histological examination shows thrombi consisting of fibrin and platelets in the terminal interlobular arteries, the afferent arterioles and glomerular capillaries.

Treatment involves corticosteroid therapy and plasma exchange.

Renal infarction

Embolic infarction
The embolus can come from:

- Thrombotic material from the left side of the heart
- Atheromatous material from plaques
- Bacterial vegetations from infective endocarditis.

The emboli lodge in the small renal vessels and cause narrowing of the arterioles and focal areas of ischaemic injury. It can be asymptomatic, or present with haematuria and loin tenderness. The areas of infarction appear pale and are characteristically wedge shaped.

Diffuse cortical necrosis
Diffuse cortical necrosis causes ARF and presents with anuria. This is a rare condition that results from profound hypertension caused by:

- Severe hypovolaemic shock
- Sepsis
- Eclampsia (pregnancy).

In response to hypotension, there is compensatory vasoconstriction that can cause infarction. This can be avoided by prompt resuscitation of the shocked patient. Once the disease is established, no agent has been shown to improve outcome. Prognosis is much better for focal infarction than for generalized cortical infarction. The surface of the kidney appears patchy with irregular yellow areas of necrosis, congestion and haemorrhage (limited to the outer part of the cortex). Infarcts can calcify over time.

Sickle-cell disease nephropathy

Thrombotic occlusion by deformed sickle-shaped red cells causes papillary necrosis. It is precipitated by cold, dehydration, infection and exercise. Presentation is with pain, haematuria and polyuria. Management involves analgesia, warmth and rehydration, blood transfusions and antibiotics (if infection is suspected).

NEOPLASTIC DISEASE OF THE KIDNEY

Benign tumours of the kidney

These rarely cause symptoms and are usually found on autopsy as an incidental finding.

Renal fibroma or hamartoma

This is the most common benign renal tumour. It is a small (less than 1 cm diameter) firm, well-demarcated, white nodule in the medulla. The nodule is composed of spindle cells and collagen. It is often an incidental finding with clinical significance.

Cortical adenoma

This is a small (<3 cm diameter) discrete, yellowish-grey tumour derived from renal tubular epithelium. It is an incidental finding in 20–25% of autopsies; it has a low malignant potential. On histological examination it is found to be composed of large vacuolated clear cells with small nuclei (this is also seen in renal cell carcinoma). Diagnosis depends on the size of the tumour:

- Less than 30 mm diameter: benign adenoma
- Over 30 mm diameter: malignant carcinoma

However, this grading is unreliable because small lesions could be growing carcinomas.

Angiomyolipoma (hamartomatous malformation)

This is found in the cortex or medulla. The tumour is composed of blood vessels, smooth muscle and fat. Angiomyolipomas are associated with tuberous sclerosis, which is an inherited disease that involves the CNS, skin and other viscera.

Oncocytoma

This is an epithelial cell tumour that can grow to a diameter of 12 cm but does not undergo malignant change. Histological examination reveals enlarged cells with a granular eosinophilic cytoplasm as a result of the vast number of mitochondria in the tumour cells.

Malignant tumours of the kidney

Renal cell carcinoma

Incidence and risk factors

Approximately 90% of renal malignant tumours in adults are renal cell carcinomas (RCCs), which arise from the tubular epithelium. RCCs are rare in children and have a peak incidence in 60–70-year-olds. The male to female ratio is 3:1. There is great geographical variance with the highest incidence in Scandinavia and the lowest in South America and Africa. Risk factors are:

- Acquired cystic disease in patients who require renal replacement therapy – RCC tends to occur at a much earlier age in these patients.
- Von Hippel–Lindau disease: this is a rare autosomal dominant condition caused by a mutation on chromosome 25; 50–70% of these patients develop RCC.
- Smoking.

Presentation

Approximately 90% of cases present with haematuria. Non-specific symptoms include fatigue, weight loss and fever. There might be a mass in the loin. These are all late manifestations, presenting at an advanced stage of tumour progression, which is why prognosis is poor. RCCs often metastasize before local symptoms develop.

A small number of RCCs can secrete hormone-like substances such as:

- Parathyroid hormone, resulting in hypercalcaemia
- Adrenocorticotrophic hormone (ACTH), resulting in a Cushing's-like syndrome
- Erythropoietin, resulting in polycythaemia
- Renin, resulting in hypertension.

As a result of these hormone-producing tumours, RCC commonly presents with paraneoplastic syndromes.

Diagnosis
Diagnosis is by:

- IVU: this reveals a space-occupying lesion in the kidney that distorts the outline.
- Ultrasonography: this distinguishes between solid and cystic lesions.
- CT: provides preoperative staging (see Chapter 8).

Pathology
RCC consists of a yellow-brown, well-demarcated mass in the renal cortex, with a diameter of 3–15 cm.

Within this area there are patches of haemorrhage, necrosis and cyst formation. The tumours are most common at the upper pole of the kidney. The renal capsule is often intact, although it can be breached and the tumour will extend into the perinephric fat. Spread into the renal vein is often visible and rarely this extends into the inferior vena cava.

Histological examination reveals cells with clear cytoplasm that range from well differentiated to anaplastic.

Spread occurs by direct invasion of local tissues, via the lymph to lumbar nodes (a third of cases), and via the blood (venous). Metastases are found in the lung, liver, bone, opposite kidney and adrenals.

Prognosis
Prognosis depends on tumour size and the degree of the spread; RCC staging involves assessing local, nodal and metastatic spread (TNM classification).

T_1: confined to the kidney
T_2: enlarging tumour with distortion of the kidney with renal capsule intact
T_3: spread through the renal capsule into the perinephric fat with invasion into the renal vein
T_4: invasion into adjacent organs or the abdominal wall
N^+: lymph node involvement
M^+: metastatic spread.

Treatment
If there are no distant metastases, treatment involves a radical nephrectomy with removal of the associated adrenal gland, perinephric fat, upper ureter and the para-aortic lymph nodes. Postoperative radiotherapy is required to decrease risk of recurrence. There is little effective treatment available for metastatic disease. The average 5-year survival rate is 45%, increasing up to 70% if there is no metastatic disease at diagnosis.

Wilms' tumour (nephroblastoma)

Incidence and presentation
This is the most common malignant tumour in children. The peak incidence is in 1–4-year-olds, with both sexes affected equally. It is an embryonic tumour derived from the primitive metanephros. It presents with an abdominal mass and occasionally haematuria, abdominal pain and hypertension.

Pathology
The tumours are large solid masses of firm white tissue with areas of necrosis and haemorrhage. They

often breach the renal capsule and grow into the perinephric fat. Histological examination reveals spindle cells or primitive blastema cells with epithelial and mesenchymal tissues, cartilage, bone and muscle. They are aggressive tumours, often presenting with metastatic disease of the lung.

Treatment and prognosis

Treatment involves nephrectomy, radiotherapy and chemotherapy. The long-term survival rate is over 80%.

Prognosis depends upon tumour size and distant spread at the time of diagnosis.

Urothelial carcinoma of the renal pelvis

This is a transitional cell tumour accounting for 5–10% of renal tumours. It can be caused by:

* Analgesic misuse
* Exposure to aniline dyes used in the industrial manufacture of dyes, rubber and plastics.

Presentation with haematuria or obstruction occurs early, because the renal pelvis projects directly into the pelvicalyceal cavity.

Histological picture ranges from well-differentiated tumours to diffuse, invasive and anaplastic carcinomas. Poorly differentiated tumours have a poor prognosis and often invade the wall of the renal pelvis and the renal vein. Multiple tumours are also often found in the ureters and bladder. Fragments of papillary tumour and atypical tumour cells can be detected in the urine and this makes cytological diagnosis possible.

> Metastases from lymphomas, lung or breast cancer or melanomas can deposit in the kidneys.

Figure 4.11 summarizes the common tumour sites throughout the urinary tract.

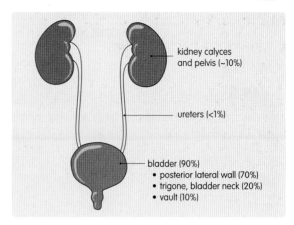

Fig. 4.11 Common tumour sites throughout the urinary tract.

kidney calyces and pelvis (~10%)

ureters (<1%)

bladder (90%)
• posterior lateral wall (70%)
• trigone, bladder neck (20%)
• vault (10%)

RENAL RESPONSES TO SYSTEMIC DISORDERS

Congestive cardiac failure

Congestive cardiac failure (CCF) occurs when the heart cannot cope with its work load (i.e. providing the body with its metabolic requirements) and the cardiac output fails to perfuse the tissues adequately. This results in hypoperfusion of tissues and sodium and water retention. CCF is the common end result of all types of severe heart disease.

> CCF can be caused by:
>
> * Pump failure (low-output heart failure)
> * Increased demand (high-output heart failure).
>
> A normal heart can fail under high loads, but an abnormal heart will fail under normal loads.
>   The kidney tries to increase fluid volume, leading to peripheral oedema, and eventually pulmonary oedema.

A fall in cardiac output leads to renal hypoperfusion. The kidney senses this as a sign of hypovolaemia and compensates by retaining NaCl and water to increase the circulating volume (Fig. 4.12). As the kidney attempts to increase the circulating fluid volume, peripheral oedema develops (left heart failure). This increases pulmonary venous pressure, resulting in fluid transudation from the capillaries in the lungs, and in pulmonary oedema.

Treatment and management

Management involves reducing the fluid load within the body and thereby decreasing the workload of the heart.

* Diuretics: produce symptomatic relief from pulmonary oedema.

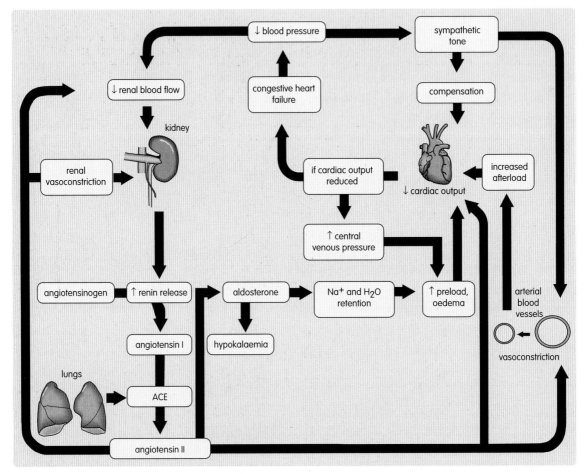

Fig. 4.12 Compensatory mechanisms in congestive cardiac failure. ACE, angiotensin-converting enzyme.

- ACE inhibitors: act as vasodilators (by reducing the synthesis of angiotensin II) and as diuretics (by decreasing aldosterone synthesis).
- Nitrates: produce venodilation, which decreases preload.
- Vasodilators (e.g. hydralazine): these reduce afterload.

Prognosis depends on the overall clinical picture, and the extent of cardiovascular disease. For further information see *Crash course: Cardiovascular system*.

Hypovolaemia and shock

Shock is a medical emergency in which the vital organs are hypoperfused as a result of either an inadequate circulating blood volume or heart failure. As the amount of oxygen and nutrients delivered to the cells is inadequate, the resulting hypoxic state within the cells leads to anaerobic metabolism and there is inefficient clearance of the metabolites, which build up in the cell. Hypovolaemia and mild shock cause tiredness, dizziness and a feeling of thirst. A severe decrease in the circulating volume stimulates sympathetic activity to maintain the blood pressure by:

- Tachycardia
- Peripheral vasoconstriction
- Increase in myocardial contractility.

Vasodilation occurs in the vital organs (heart, lungs, brain) to maintain blood supply, but this is at the expense of perfusion to other organs. If there is inadequate compensation, tissue hypoxia and necrosis can occur in vulnerable organs (e.g. acute tubular necrosis in the kidneys).

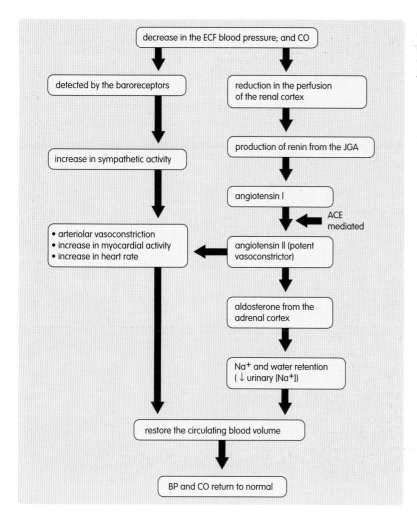

Fig. 4.13 Response to a fall in circulating fluid volume. ACE, angiotensin-converting enzyme; BP, blood pressure; CO, cardiac output; ECF, extracellular fluid; JGA, juxtaglomerular apparatus.

Types of shock

Cardiogenic shock

This occurs when the heart fails to maintain cardiac output acutely (e.g. ischaemic heart disease, arrhythmias). As a result, tissue perfusion decreases dramatically. Venous pressure increases, causing pulmonary or peripheral oedema (as described above). Prognosis is poor (90% mortality).

Hypovolaemic shock

This occurs when there is an acute reduction in effective circulating blood volume:

- Exogenous losses of plasma (e.g. burns), of blood (e.g. haemorrhage), or of water and electrolytes (e.g. diarrhoea and vomiting)
- Endogenous losses of fluid (e.g. sepsis and anaphylaxis).

Figure 4.13 shows the response to a fall in circulating fluid volume. To avoid excessive sympathetic activity in the kidneys (this results in vasoconstriction), more vasodilating prostaglandins (PGE_2 and PGI_2) are secreted within the kidneys. This maintains adequate blood flow through the kidney to allow sufficient glomerular filtration, unless the shock is severe. The loss of large amounts of fluid has two major consequences:

- Volume depletion (decreases tissue perfusion)
- Electrolyte and acid–base disturbance.

As Na^+ is involved in the co-transport of H^+, K^+ and Cl^-, the acid–base balance is disturbed because Na^+ is retained. Cl^- is reabsorbed in equal quantities but, initially, there is increased secretion of H^+ and K^+, resulting in metabolic alkalosis (contraction alkalosis) and hypokalaemia. This is balanced by the shift to anaerobic metabolism as a result of hypoxia in the tissues, which eventually prevails to cause a metabolic acidosis. This is further potentiated as hypovolaemia becomes more severe, as less urine is excreted and H^+ is no longer excreted.

Treatment

Treatment of cardiogenic shock involves inotropes, whereas treatment of hypovolaemic shock requires fluid replacement to restore the extracellular volume. HCO_3^- is considered if there is severe acidosis (pH <7.2) (see p. 57 for acid-base disturbances). If blood flow to the kidneys is not restored, renal failure results from tissue anoxia and necrosis.

Hypertension

Blood pressure (BP) is influenced by the interaction of genetic and environmental factors, which regulate cardiac output (CO) and total peripheral resistance (TPR):

$$BP = CO \times TPR$$

The kidneys influence blood pressure by regulating the volume of extracellular fluid (ECF). They also release vasoactive substances:

- Vasoconstrictors: angiotensin II
- Vasodilators: prostaglandins.

Renal autoregulation maintains renal function despite variations in systolic blood pressure. Any change in the ECF will affect the blood pressure. The kidney compensates for these changes by controlling Na^+ and water excretion. If this mechanism is disturbed there will be uncontrolled Na^+ and water retention, resulting in hypertension. Hypertension is defined by the World Health Organization as a sustained blood pressure of 140/90 mmHg or above.

Essential hypertension

This accounts for about 95% of all cases of hypertension and the cause is unknown. Initially, there is an increase in cardiac output as a result of sympathetic overactivity. In the later stages the increase in blood pressure is maintained by an increase in the total peripheral resistance, but cardiac output is normal. Hypertensive changes seen in the kidney include:

- Arteriosclerosis of the major renal arteries (RAS)
- Hyalinization of the small vessels with intimal thickening.

This can lead to chronic renal damage (hypertensive nephrosclerosis) and a reduction in the size of the kidneys.

Malignant or 'accelerated' hypertension is a rare and rapidly progressing form of severe hypertension. It is characterized by fibrinoid necrosis of the blood vessel walls, and ischaemic damage to the brain and kidney. This can lead to acute renal failure or heart failure, requiring urgent treatment.

Secondary hypertension

This is caused by renal (80%) and endocrine diseases, and occasionally drugs (ciclosporin).

Renal mechanisms causing hypertension include:

- Impaired sodium and water excretion, increasing blood volume
- Stimulation of renin release.

The kidneys influence blood pressure by regulating ECF volume, and also release vasoactive substances:

- Vasoconstrictors: angiotensin II
- Vasodilators: prostaglandins.

Renal artery stenosis

This accounts for up to half of renal-induced hypertension cases. There are two types:

- Atherosclerosis: common (see above). Renal impairment is frequent and there is only a variable or incomplete improvement in hypertension with treatment
- Fibromuscular dysplasia: rare (seen in young women) (see Fig. 4.10). Renal impairment is unusual and hypertension often cured by treatment.

Narrowing of the renal vessels reduces the pressure in the afferent arterioles, which stimulates the juxtaglomerular apparatus to secrete renin. This increases plasma angiotensin II, which causes vasoconstriction and aldosterone release. Aldosterone promotes Na^+ and therefore fluid retention (this increases BP), and increases K^+ secretion.

Intrinsic renal diseases

These account for over half of renal induced hypertension and include any cause of chronic GN, chronic pyelonephritis and polycystic kidney disease.

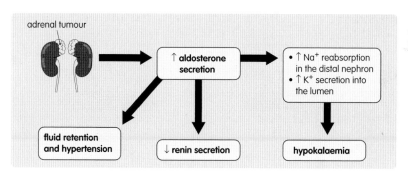

Patients with primary glomerular disease present with hypertension – which is more severe – earlier than patients with renal interstitial disease.

Endocrine causes

The endocrine causes are:

- Cushing's syndrome
- Oestrogen (i.e. the contraceptive pill and pregnancy)
- Phaeochromocytoma (rare)
- Primary hyperaldosteronism (Conn's syndrome).

In primary hyperaldosteronism there is chronic excessive secretion of aldosterone because of an adrenal cortical adenoma or hyperplasia (Fig. 4.14). Patients present with hypertension and hypokalaemia. Diagnosis is made based on the triad of:

- Hypokalaemia
- Increased aldosterone
- Decreased renin.

Treatment is by surgical removal of the adenoma, with a cure rate of 60% or aldosterone antagonists (spironolactone). Recent studies have suggested that hyperaldosteronism may be a more common cause of hypertension than previously realized.

Management of hypertension

It is difficult to detect and treat hypertension because it is often asymptomatic, and many patients are reluctant to take medication if they feel well. It is very important to exclude an underlying cause of hypertension.

Hypertension is an important risk factor for strokes, cardiac failure, myocardial infarction and renal failure. Effective treatment will improve the prognosis for each of these conditions.

Lifestyle changes include:

- Weight reduction
- Reduced alcohol intake
- Salt restriction
- Regular exercise
- Smoking cessation.

Drug treatment of hypertension involves:

- Diuretics (i.e. loop diuretics and thiazide diuretics – see p. 92)
- ACE inhibitors
- β-blockers
- Vasodilators (i.e. Ca^{2+} channel blockers).

Angiotensin-converting enzyme inhibitors

These inhibit ACE, and so block formation of angiotensin II. Angiotensin II is a potent vasoconstrictor and promotes sodium reabsorption in the tubule. This system is stimulated by:

- Renal arteriolar pressure
- Sympathetic stimulation
- Reduced delivery of sodium to the distal tubule (Fig. 4.15).

ACE inhibitors (e.g. captopril, ramipril) lower blood pressure by:

- Reducing total peripheral resistance
- Inhibiting the local (tissue) renin–angiotensin system.

ACE inhibitors also reduce proteinuria and delay the progress of renal disease in patients with diabetic nephropathy and patients with proteinuric non-diabetic renal disease. They are also used to treat CCF.

Fig. 4.15 Effects of ACE (angiotensin-converting enzyme) inhibitors. +ve, positive feedback; –ve, negative feedback.

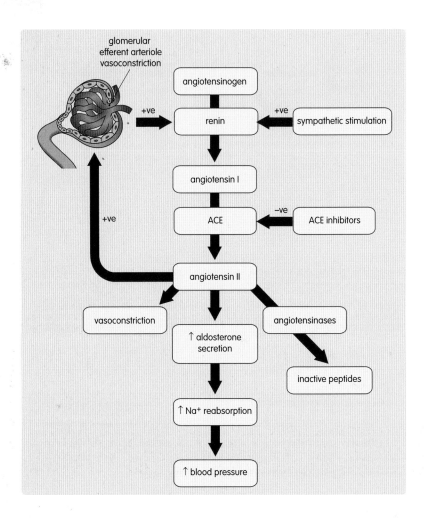

The side-effects of ACE inhibitors include:

- Persistent dry cough
- Allergic reactions or rashes
- Dose-related proteinuria (rare)
- Changes in the sensation of taste
- Severe hypotension especially in patients who are hypovolaemic
- Acute renal failure in patients with RAS (renal function should be checked after giving ACE inhibitors)
- Hyperkalaemia.

ACE inhibitors are contraindicated in the final two trimesters of pregnancy because of the risk of:

- Developmental abnormalities in the fetal kidney
- Oligohydramnios (reduced amniotic fluid)
- Neonatal hypotension and anuria.

Renal causes of hypertension are:

- RAS (renovascular hypertension)
- Intrinsic renal disease (renal hypertension)
- Primary hyperaldosteronism (causing renal Na^+ retention and K^+ excretion)
- Excess renin production (e.g. renal tumour).

Hepatorenal syndrome

Patients with liver disease can have a reduced urine flow (oliguria). This is especially so in patients with portal hypertension and ascites. Portal hypertension results from an increase in resistance to blood flow from the gut and spleen, resulting in venous congestion due to nitric oxide release. This stimulates renin release. As there appears to be a fall in arterial blood volume, Na^+ and water are retained. As a result of increased resistance in the liver caused by hepatic cirrhosis, hydrostatic pressure in the portal vein increases. This causes fluid to accumulate in the peritoneal cavity (ascites) as fluid is forced out of the interstitial capillaries. This further reduces the circulating blood volume, which again stimulates renin release. Thus, a positive feedback loop promoting hypertension is set up.

Liver disease can also impair albumin synthesis. This decreases the oncotic (colloid osmotic) pressure in the capillaries, favouring fluid movement out and worsening the ascites. Circulating blood volume is further reduced.

A major complication of nephrotic syndrome is renal vein thrombosis, which should be suspected if proteinuria increases or renal function deteriorates. Diagnosis is by ultrasound, and treatment involves anticoagulation.

INTERVENTIONS IN RENAL DISEASE

Medical management of renal disease

Diuretics

Diuretics increase the volume of urine produced by increasing renal sodium excretion (natriuresis), which is followed passively by water. Each type of diuretic has specific actions on the normal physiology of a particular segment (Fig. 4.16):

- Act on the membrane transport proteins found on the luminal surface
- Interfere with hormone receptors
- Inhibit enzyme activity.

Osmotic diuretics

Osmotic diuresis can be induced by an inert substance that is not reabsorbed in the tubule. The proximal tubule and the descending limb of the loop of Henle allow free movement of water molecules. If an agent such as mannitol is introduced into the tubular fluid, it is not absorbed and thus reduces water reabsorption. There is increased

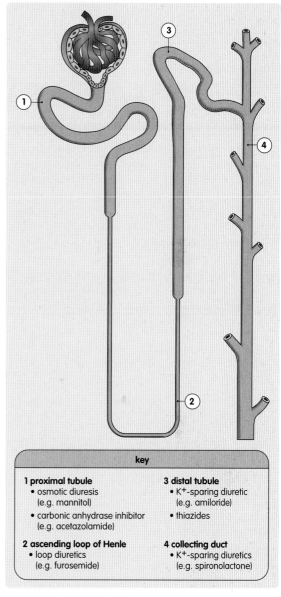

key

1 proximal tubule
- osmotic diuresis (e.g. mannitol)
- carbonic anhydrase inhibitor (e.g. acetazolamide)

2 ascending loop of Henle
- loop diuretics (e.g. furosemide)

3 distal tubule
- K^+-sparing diuretic (e.g. amiloride)
- thiazides

4 collecting duct
- K^+-sparing diuretics (e.g. spironolactone)

Fig. 4.16 Sites of diuretic action.

urine flow through the nephrons resulting in reduced sodium reabsorption.

Osmotic diuretics are used to:

- Increase urine volume when renal haemodynamics are compromised, and thus prevent anuria
- Reduce intracranial pressures in neurological conditions
- Reduce intraocular pressures before ophthalmic surgery.

Excessive use of osmotic diuretics without adequate fluid replacement can cause dehydration and hypernatraemia.

Loop diuretics

These are the most powerful diuretics, causing up to 20% of filtered Na^+ to be excreted. They inhibit sodium transport out of the thick ascending limb of the loop of Henle into the medullary interstitium. Examples include furosemide and bumetanide. Loop diuretics (e.g. furosemide) act by inhibiting the $Na^+/K^+/2Cl^-$ co-transporter on the luminal membrane of the cells. This inhibits Na^+ reabsorption, thereby diluting the osmotic gradient in the medulla. This results in increased Na^+ and water excretion. Positive lumen potential falls as cations are retained, causing an increase in Ca^{2+} and Mg^{2+} excretion. As a higher $[Na^+]$ reaches the distal tubule, there is increased K^+ secretion, so loop diuretics can be used to reduce total body K^+.

Loop diuretics are used for:

- Acute pulmonary and peripheral oedema
- To reduce end-diastolic ventricular filling pressure
- Pulmonary congestion
- Acute hypercalcaemia
- Hypertension
- Nephrotic syndrome
- Acute renal failure (increases urine output and K^+ excretion).

The side-effects of loop diuretics include:

- Hypokalaemic metabolic alkalosis
- Hypovolaemia and hypotension
- Hyperuricaemia (can precipitate attacks of gout)
- Hypomagnesaemia
- Ototoxicity (dose-related reversible auditory loss)
- Allergic reactions.

Thiazide diuretics

These reduce active Na^+ reabsorption in the early distal tubule by inhibiting the Na^+/Cl^- co-transporter. As there is more reabsorption of Na^+ in the loop of Henle, the loop diuretics are more potent than thiazide diuretics. Thiazides help reduce peripheral vascular resistance, and consequently are used to manage hypertension. They are also used in CCF and nephrogenic diabetes insipidus.

Renal-related side-effects of thiazide diuretics include:

- Hypokalaemic metabolic alkalosis
- Hyperglycaemia

- Hyperlipidaemia
- Hyperuricaemia
- Hypercalcaemia
- Hyponatraemia.

Side-effects unrelated to renal actions include:

- Hypercholesterolaemia
- Reversible male impotence
- Allergic reactions (rare).

Side-effects of thiazide diuretics: HyperGLUC (hyper glucose, lipid, uric acid and calcium).

Potassium-sparing diuretics

These diuretics are K^+-sparing and act:

- In the collecting ducts (e.g. spironolactone)
- By inhibiting the uptake of Na^+ in the cells of the distal nephron (e.g. amiloride and triamterene).

Aldosterone is a mineralocorticoid that increases the activity of the Na^+/K^+ ATPase, potassium and sodium channels, resulting in Na^+ absorption and K^+ secretion.

Spironolactone (a mineralocorticoid analogue) competes with aldosterone for the receptor site. This reduces sodium reabsorption in the distal nephron and decreases K^+ secretion (potassium-sparing activity).

Potassium-sparing diuretics are used if there is mineralocorticoid excess such as primary aldosteronism (Conn's syndrome) or ectopic ACTH production. They are also used in secondary aldosteronism where salt and water retention have occurred (e.g. CCF, nephrotic syndrome, liver disease and hypovolaemia). They are fairly weak, often used with loop diuretics or thiazides to prevent K^+ loss.

The side-effects include:

- Hyperkalaemia: this results from an increase in H^+-and therefore K^+-retention as Na^+ absorption falls and ranges from mild to life-threatening.
- Endocrine effects with spironolactone (e.g. gynaecomastia).

Potassium-sparing diuretics are contraindicated in patients with chronic renal insufficiency.

Carbonic anhydrase inhibitors

Carbonic anhydrase (CA) is found in many places in the nephron but primarily on the brush border of the luminal membrane of the proximal tubule cells. CA catalyses the dehydration of H_2CO_3:

$$H^+ + HCO_3^- \rightleftharpoons H_2CO_3 \rightleftharpoons H_2O + CO_2$$

This reaction is driven by H^+ secretion into the lumen, by cotransport with Na^+. Once in the cell, H_2CO_3 is reformed under the influence of intracellular CA, the HCO_3^- ions are reabsorbed, and H^+ is secreted back into the lumen (see Fig. 2.23).

CA inhibitors interfere with the action of carbonic anhydrase and inhibit HCO_3^- reabsorption. The presence of HCO_3^- in the lumen reduces Na^+ reabsorption, which continues into the distal nephron where it enhances K^+ secretion.

CA inhibitors such as acetazolamide are weak diuretics, which cause the excretion of only about 5–10% of the filtered Na^+ and water. Their main clinical use is to treat acute and chronic glaucoma by reducing intraocular pressure (the production of aqueous humour in the eye involves secretion of HCO_3^- by the ciliary body in a process similar to that in the proximal tubule).

The side-effects of CA inhibitors include:

- Metabolic acidosis
- Renal stones
- Renal K^+ wasting
- Nervous system effects – paraesthesia and drowsiness.

CA inhibitors should be avoided in patients with liver disease or advanced CRF.

A summary of the main classes of diuretic is shown in Figure 4.17.

Dialysis and haemofiltration

Dialysis imitates the kidney by temporarily removing waste products and excess fluids that accumulate in renal failure. It is used to treat renal failure in patients with acute or chronic renal failure. Indications for dialysis include:

- GFR <5–10 mL/min
- Blood urea >30 mmol/L
- Hyperkalaemia
- Acidosis
- Fluid overload.

A semi-permeable membrane acts as a filter, with a dialysate solution to regulate the fluid and electrolytes in the blood. There are three forms of dialysis: haemodialysis, haemofiltration and continuous ambulatory peritoneal dialysis (Fig. 4.18). At best, it provides an equivalent average clearance of approximately 10 mL/min (normal GFR 120 mL/min).

Haemodialysis

This involves pumping the blood through an artificial kidney, called a dialysis machine. Blood flows on one side of a semi-permeable membrane,

Fig. 4.17 Summary of the three main classes of diuretics	Loop diuretics	Thiazide diuretics	K⁺-sparing diuretics
diuretic capability	+++	++	+
site of action	thick ascending loop of Henle	distal tubule	collecting tubule
mechanism of action	inhibit Na⁺/K⁺/2Cl co-transporter, and thus increase Na⁺ and K⁺ loss	inhibit the Na⁺/Cl co-transporter (K⁺ loss, Ca²⁺ loss)	block Na⁺ channels and thus antagonize aldosterone receptors
side-effects	hypokalaemia; metabolic acidosis; hypovolaemia	hypokalaemia; metabolic alkalosis	hyperkalaemia
example	furosemide	bendroflumethiazide	spironolactone; amiloride

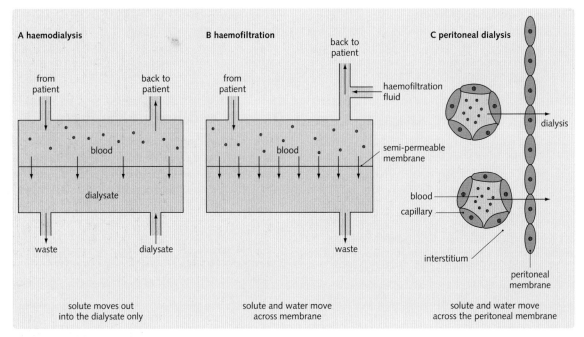

Fig. 4.18 Comparison of the three different methods of dialysis. (A) haemodialysis; (B) haemofiltration and (C) peritoneal dialysis (adapted from O'Callaghan CA, Bremmer BM 2001 The kidney at a glance. Blackwell Science, pp. 96, 98).

with dialysis fluid being passed in the opposite direction on the other side. Typically, blood flows at 300 mL/min and the dialysate fluid flows at 500 mL/min. Dialysis occurs across the semi-permeable membrane removing toxins from the blood down a concentration gradient.

Several synthetic semi-permeable membranes are available, with different permeability characteristics. The dialysate is made of purified water with a solute composition similar to plasma, but without any of the waste products, so solutes move along their concentration gradient out of the blood.

Access to the circulation is gained by an arterio-venous (AV) fistula, which is constructed surgically, usually by joining the radial artery and cephalic vein. The venous system 'arterializes' and the high blood flows required for dialysis can be obtained by 'needling' the venous system. Complications of the AV fistula include infection and thrombosis.

Dialysis 'dose' can be adjusted by altering the blood flow, the area of the semi-permeable membrane, or the duration of treatment. On average, patients require approximately 4 h of treatment three times a week.

Complications of haemodialysis include:

- Hypotension
- Infection
- Haemolysis
- Air embolism
- Reactions to dialysis membrane.

Haemofiltration

This involves filtering blood across a semi-permeable membrane allowing removal of small molecules. The fluid is replaced with that of the appropriate biochemical composition. The replacement fluid is commonly buffered by lactate. Haemofiltration is used predominantly for the treatment of ARF, especially in the intensive care unit setting. When performed slowly (continuous veno-veno haemofiltration), it causes smaller fluid shifts and therefore less hypotension than haemodialysis.

Both haemodialysis and haemofiltration can be used continuously in ARF to ensure slow continuous correction of the fluid and electrolyte balance, especially in patients with haemodynamic instability.

Continuous ambulatory peritoneal dialysis

Continuous ambulatory peritoneal dialysis (CAPD) uses the peritoneal membrane as the semi-permeable membrane. Unlike haemodialysis, peritoneal dialysis does not require an AV fistula for circulatory access. Instead, it requires the insertion of a permanent 'Tenchkoff' catheter through the anterior abdominal wall into the peritoneal cavity. Dialysate solution is introduced into the peritoneum and exchanged regularly for fresh fluid – up to five times a day is necessary to maintain the efficiency of dialysis. Waste products pass into the dialysate along their concentration gradients and water is removed by osmosis. Dialysis solutions with high osmolarity will remove more water. Dextrose is commonly used to induce osmosis, but is gradually absorbed by the patient. Newer, non-absorbable, osmotic agents are now available (e.g. glucose polymer). CAPD is used in the maintenance dialysis of end-stage renal failure, but technique survival declines to 50% after 5 years due to loss of peritoneal membrane function.

Complications of peritoneal dialysis include:

- Peritonitis (50% is caused by *Staphylococcus epidermidis*). Treatment is with intraperitoneal or intravenous antibiotics
- Mechanical problems with fluid drainage
- Infections or blockage around the site of the catheter
- Other complications include pleural effusions and sclerosing peritonitis (rare but serious).

Contraindications to CAPD are:

- Peritoneal adhesions as a result of peritonitis
- Abdominal hernia
- Colostomy.

> Dialysis is essential in patients presenting with hyperkalaemia, acidosis, pulmonary oedema and uraemic complications. Complications include hypotension, infection and haemolysis.

Renal transplantation

This is the most successful organ transplantation and is the ideal treatment for end-stage irreversible renal failure. It restores near-normal renal function and improves quality of life. The kidney may come

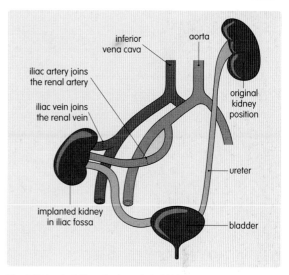

Fig. 4.19 Implantation of a transplanted kidney.

from a cadaver, a close living relative or a partner and is usually placed in the iliac fossa. The renal vessels from the donated kidney are anastomosed onto the iliac blood vessels of the recipient and the ureter is inserted into the bladder (Fig. 4.19). Success depends upon:

- ABO group
- Matching the donor and the recipient for HLA types
- Preoperative blood transfusion
- Immunosuppressive treatment.

Short-term complications include:

- Acute rejection (within 3 months)
- Operative failure.

Rejection is reduced by immunosuppression therapy, which is started after the transplantation and continued indefinitely. However, patients are at risk of opportunistic infection (e.g. with cytomegalovirus). Long-term complications include:

- Infection
- Recurrence of original disease
- Obstruction at the ureteric anastomoses
- Malignancy, especially lymphomas.

Currently, the 1-year graft survival rate is in excess of 80% for cadaveric transplants and 90% for live donor transplants.

By the end of the chapter you should be able to:

- Explain what the 'trigone' is and how it differs from the rest of the bladder
- Explain the differences between the external and internal urethral sphincters
- Outline the function of the detrusor and sphincter muscles, and their innervation
- Summarize common neurological causes of difficulties with micturition
- Describe the effects of 'spinal shock'
- Understand the difference between a hydroureter and a megaloureter
- Explain how diverticula develop, where they occur and their long-term effects
- Name three causes of urinary tract obstruction and list the imaging techniques you would use to investigate obstruction
- Describe how clinical presentation of urinary obstruction is influenced by the site and cause of the obstruction
- Discuss how bilateral hydronephrosis differs in presentation from unilateral hydronephrosis
- Summarize the factors influencing stone formation and outline their management
- Outline the mechanism by which schistosomiasis increases the risk of bladder cancer
- Understand the causes of inflammation of the prostate
- Define benign prostatic hyperplasia and explain the histological changes
- Explain how treatment and prognosis differ according to the stage of prostate cancer.

ORGANIZATION OF THE LOWER URINARY TRACT

Macroscopic organization

Overview

Urine formed in the kidneys collects in the renal pelvis and then passes down the lower urinary tract (ureters, bladder and urethra) before exiting the body. The bladder stores the urine, which is ejected intermittently from the body under voluntary control.

Ureters

The ureters are hollow muscular tubes 25–30 cm long, which begin as funnel-shaped tubes at the renal pelvis. They run retroperitoneally over the posterior abdominal wall in front of the external iliac artery down to the pelvic brim (similar course in the female). Figures 5.1 and 5.2 show the course of the ureters through the pelvis in a man and woman, respectively. As urine collects in the renal pelvis, the pelvis dilates. Action potentials in the pacemaker cells of the renal pelvis are set up, stimulating peristaltic contractions in the ureters that propel the urine.

The ureters are divided into regions related to their anatomical course: renal pelvis, abdominal, pelvic and intramural regions (Fig. 5.3). This influences the source of blood supply to each region of the ureter-renal, lumbar segmental, gonadal, common iliac, internal iliac and superior vesical arteries, with corresponding venous drainage.

The ureters are innervated by both sympathetic and parasympathetic nerves. Sensory nerves are from T11–L2 and S2–4, but the motor supply to the muscular wall is unclear. As shown in Figure 5.3 there are constrictions in the ureters. Stones can get stuck at these constrictions and produce acute colicky pain, which is referred to the skin of T11–L2. Therefore, pain starts in the loin and radiates to the scrotum and penis (men) or to the labium majus (women).

Fig. 5.1 Anatomy of the male lower urinary tract.

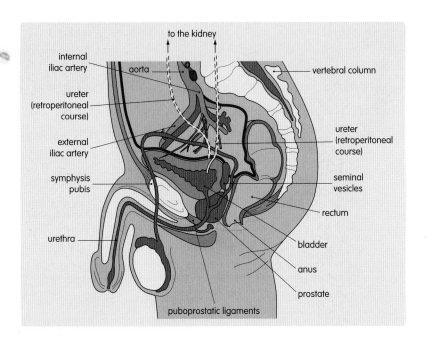

Fig. 5.2 Anatomy of the female lower urinary tract.

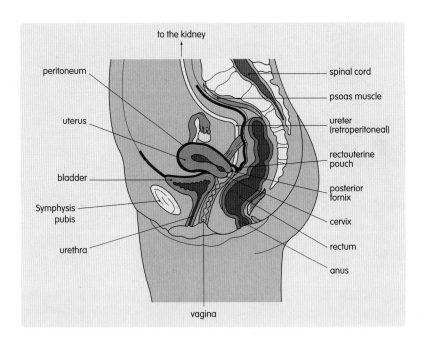

Lymphatic drainage is to the para-aortic lymph nodes.

Reflux of urine from the bladder back into the ureter is prevented by a valvular mechanism at the vesicoureteric junction. If the valve is incompetent, urinary reflux occurs and acute pyelonephritis ensues.

Urinary bladder

The ureters enter the base of the bladder, which is partially covered by peritoneum.

- When empty, it lies in the pelvis and rests on the symphysis pubis and floor of the pelvis.
- When filled, it enlarges into the abdominal cavity.

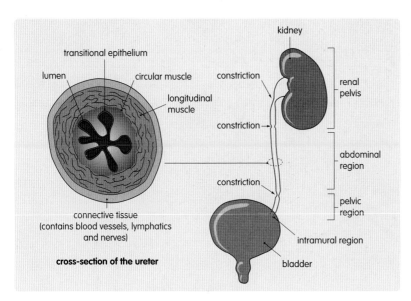

Fig. 5.3 Regions of the ureter and cross-sectional view. The normal points of reduced diameter are also shown, at which stones commonly lodge.

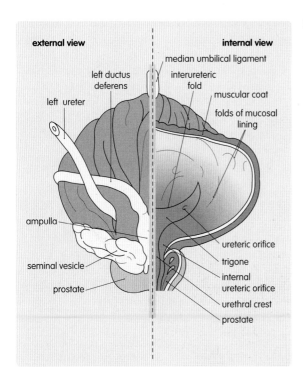

Fig. 5.4 Posterior and interior view of the male bladder.

The neck of the bladder is relatively immobile and fixed by the puboprostatic and lateral vesical ligament. Figure 5.4 shows the internal and external aspects of the male bladder and Figure 5.2 shows the urinary bladder in the female. The blood supply to the bladder is from the superior and inferior vesical branches of the internal iliac artery. It is drained by the vesical plexus and by the prostatic venous plexus in the male, which then drain into the internal iliac vein. Lymphatic drainage is also along the vesical blood vessels to the internal iliac nodes, then the para-aortic nodes.

Interior of the bladder

The wall is yellow with rugae (folds) allowing expansion with little increase in internal pressure.

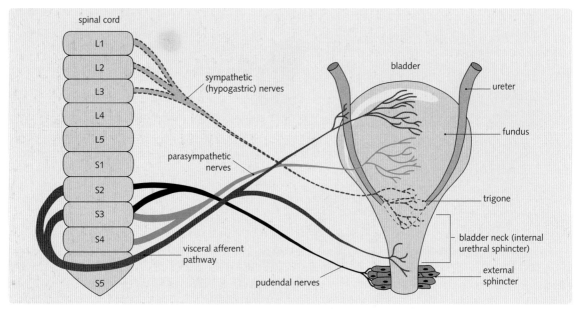

Fig. 5.5 Innervation of the bladder (from Koeppen BM, Stanton B 1996 Renal physiology, 2nd edn. Mosby Year Book).

The base is the trigone, which is a triangular, reddish region bounded by the ureteric openings into the bladder and the internal urethral meatus (see Fig. 5.4). This area is less mobile and less distensible than the rest of the bladder. It is more sensitive to painful stimuli.

The bladder is lined by smooth muscle, known as the detrusor muscle, which, like the ureter, is arranged in spiral, long and circular bundles. Smooth muscle bundles surround the bladder neck to form the internal urethral sphincter, which is under involuntary control. Slightly further along the urethra there is a skeletal muscle sphincter – the external urethral sphincter. This is under voluntary control.

- The internal urethral sphincter is not under voluntary control and thus contracts reflexly.
- The external urethral sphincter is under voluntary control.

Bladder innervation (Fig. 5.5) is both:

- **Sensory**: gives sensation (awareness) of a full bladder and also pain from disease. The impulses are suppressed if the bladder is empty.

- **Motor**: parasympathetic activity stimulates the detrusor muscle, so the bladder contracts. It also inhibits the external urethral sphincter, which relaxes to allow micturition. Sympathetic activity inhibits the detrusor muscle, so the bladder relaxes, and stimulates the urethral sphincter (this contracts). Both these actions prevent micturition.

Male urethra

The male urethra (Fig. 5.6) is longer than the female urethra (male = 20 cm, female = 4 cm). It runs through the neck of the bladder, the prostate gland, the floor of pelvis and the perineal membrane to the penis and external urethral orifice at the tip of the glans penis. It has three parts:

1. Prostatic urethra: surrounded by prostate tissue
2. Membranous urethra: the shortest region, with sphincter activity
3. Spongy urethra: surrounded by penile tissue.

It is innervated by the prostatic plexus and lymphatic drainage is to the internal iliac and deep inguinal nodes.

Female urethra

This starts at the neck of the bladder and passes through the floor of the pelvis and perineal

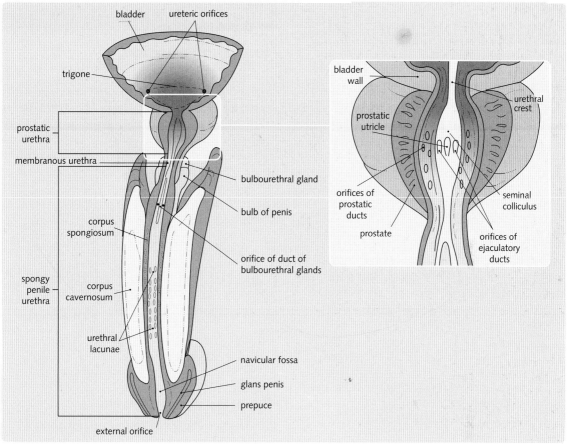

Fig. 5.6 The male urethra.

membrane to open into the vestibule just anterior to the opening of the vagina. It is 4 cm in length and is firmly attached to the anterior wall of the vagina. Lymphatics drain to the internal and external iliac lymph nodes.

Prostate

This is a gland lying below the bladder in the male and surrounding the proximal part of the urethra (prostatic urethra). It measures $4 \times 3 \times 2$ cm and is conical in shape. It is connected to the bladder by connective tissue stroma and has three parts:

1. Left lateral lobe
2. Right lateral lobe
3. Middle lobe.

The prostate has a connective tissue capsule, which is surrounded by a thick sheath from the pelvic fascia. It is influenced by sex hormones resulting in growth during puberty. From the fourth decade onwards, it hypertrophies and nodules of hyperplastic glandular and connective tissue form. As the prostate surrounds the urethra, any enlargement can narrow the urethra and obstruct urine flow.

The prostate is supplied by the inferior vesical artery and blood drains via the prostatic plexus to the vesical plexus and internal iliac vein. Lymphatics drain to the internal iliac and sacral nodes. The prostatic plexus innervates the prostate.

Microstructure of the distal urinary tract

Ureters

The muscular layers are made of smooth muscle (see Fig. 5.3) arranged in layers:

- A longitudinal layer just outside the lumen
- A middle circular layer
- Another longitudinal layer.

The lumen is lined by urinary epithelium (also known as urothelium or transitional epithelium), which is folded in the relaxed state, allowing the ureter to dilate during the passage of urine.

Urothelium (transitional epithelium)

The plasma membranes of urothelium are thicker than other cell membranes, preventing interstitial fluid from entering the concentrated urine. Urothelium is impermeable to urine. The cells have highly interdigitating cell junctions, allowing the epithelium to stretch without damaging the surfaces of the cells.

Bladder

This is similar to that of the lower third of the ureter, with smooth muscle walls and transitional epithelium.

Urethra (male and female)

In males:

- The prostatic urethra is lined by urothelium
- The rest is lined by stratified or pseudostratified columnar epithelium
- The external opening is lined by stratified squamous epithelium.

In females:

- Proximally, the urethra is lined by urothelium
- Distally and at the external opening, the urethra is lined by stratified squamous epithelium.

Prostate

The prostate contains a central zone of mucosal glands originating prenatally from the endoderm. These drain directly into the urethra. There is also a peripheral zone of mucosal glands, derived from the mesoderm, which drains into the ducts that enter the urethral sinus. Prostatic glandular epithelium can vary from inactive low cuboidal cells to active pseudostratified columnar cells, depending on the degree of androgen stimulation from the testes. The glands secrete 75% of seminal fluid, which is thin, milky and rich in citric acid and hydrolytic enzymes (e.g. fibrinolysin). This prostatic secretion liquefies coagulated semen after deposition in the female genital tract. The prostate is covered by a stroma and capsule made of dense fibroelastic connective tissue with a smooth muscle component.

MICTURITION

Normal micturition

Micturition is the intermittent voiding of urine stored in the bladder. It is an autonomic reflex that is under voluntary control. The inside of the bladder wall is folded and can expand and accommodate fluid with little increase in pressure. However, it can accommodate only a certain volume of fluid before an increase in intravesical pressure occurs, causing an urge to micturate. Figure 5.7 shows a normal cystometrogram in which pressure rise is compared with rise in volume in the bladder.

Figure 5.5 shows the innervation of the bladder. In infants, micturition is a local spinal reflex in which the bladder empties on reaching a critical pressure. However, in adults this reflex is under voluntary control, so can be inhibited or initiated by higher centres in the brain. During micturition:

- Perineal muscles and the external urethral sphincter relax
- The detrusor muscle contracts (parasympathetic activity)
- Urine flows out of the bladder.

Bladder distension with urine stimulates bladder stretch receptors, which, in turn, stimulate the afferent limb of voiding reflex and parasympathetic fibres of the bladder, resulting in the desire to urinate. Higher-centre stimulation of the pudendal nerves keeps the external sphincter closed until it is appropriate to urinate. Figure 5.8 illustrates the voluntary control of micturition.

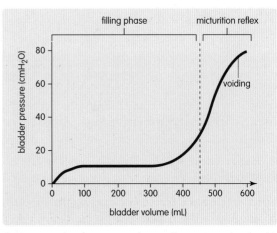

Fig. 5.7 Normal cystometrogram showing the rise in pressure associated with increasing bladder volume.

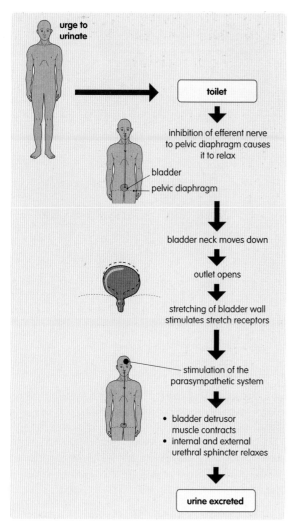

Fig. 5.8 Voluntary control of micturition.

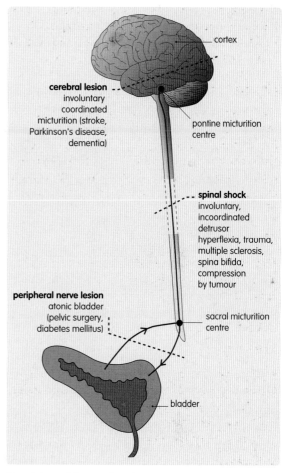

Fig. 5.9 Sites of damage along the micturition pathway.

Abnormal micturition

Neurological lesions

Urinary continence is affected by various neurological lesions along the micturition pathway, as summarized in Figure 5.9.

Lesion in the superior frontal gyrus
This can be the result of a stroke and leads to:

- Reduced desire to urinate
- Difficulty stopping micturition once started.

Lesion of afferent nerves from the bladder
A lesion of afferent nerves from the bladder (e.g. caused by disease of the dorsal roots such as tabes dorsalis) prevents reflex contractions of the bladder,

so the bladder becomes distended, thin walled and hypotonic.

Lesion of both afferent and efferent nerves
A lesion of both afferent and efferent nerves (e.g. because of a tumour of the cauda equina or filum terminale) results in:

- Initially: bladder flaccidity and distension
- Later: bladder hyperactivity with dribbling.

This leads to a shrunken bladder with a hypertrophied bladder wall.

Spinal cord lesion
A lesion to the spinal cord (e.g. spinal shock sustained following trauma) results in:

- Initially: overflow incontinence, because of a flaccid and unresponsive bladder, which results in overfill and dribbling. This is spinal shock.

103

- After shock has passed: the voiding reflex returns, but with no control from higher centres, so the patient has no voluntary control over voiding.
- Occasionally: hyperactive voiding might be seen.
- Eventually: bladder capacity falls and the wall hypertrophies – spastic neurogenic bladder.

Spinal cord injuries lead to reflex micturition, as is seen in infants. This occurs because, like infants, patients with spinal cord lesions cannot synchronize detrusor muscle contractions with sphincter relaxation.

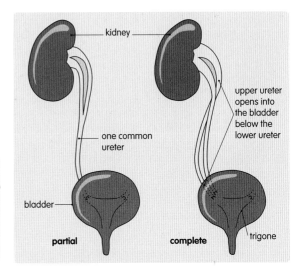

Fig. 5.10 Partial and complete bifid ureter.

Other disorders affecting micturition

Spina bifida
This is a developmental defect in which the posterior neural arches of the spine fail to develop, so part of the spinal cord and its coverings are exposed. It forms a spectrum of defects, resulting in varying degrees of bladder dysfunction.

Diabetes mellitus
Neuropathy is a common complication of diabetes. It can result in a loss of sensation, so there is no desire to micturate and the patient voids infrequently. This eventually leads to bladder distension, with overflow incontinence. The presence of residual urine increases the risk of infection.

Multiple sclerosis
This is demyelination of white matter. The bladder symptoms that develop depend on the level at which demyelination occurs.

Pelvic surgery
The nerve supply to the bladder can be injured during surgery, resulting in postoperative urinary retention. This is usually transient.

CONGENITAL ABNORMALITIES OF THE URINARY TRACT

Ureteric abnormalities
Ureteric abnormalities occur in 2–5% of the population. They are frequently bilateral and usually have no clinical relevance. Occasionally, however, they might be associated with an obstruction of urine flow.

Double and bifid ureters
The ureters along with the calyces and collecting ducts are formed from an outgrowth of the mesonephric (wolffian) duct called the ureteric bud. Early splitting of the ureteric bud or the development of two buds results in the development of double (bifid) ureters (Fig. 5.10). The duplication can be:

- Partial: the two ureters meet before entering the bladder together.
- Complete: the two ureters enter the bladder separately. The upper pole ureter enters the bladder lower and more medially than the lower ureter (see Fig. 5.10).

It is often associated with double renal pelvises with their own renal parenchyma. Renal function is rarely affected. There is a strong predisposition to infection. Urine can reflux from the bladder, especially through the upper pole ureter. Treatment involves excision of the refluxing ureter (usually the upper one).

Ureteropelvic junction obstruction
This often presents in infancy, although milder forms might not present until later in adult life or may be found in asymptomatic patients at postmortem. It is more common in males and in the left

ureter. It is bilateral in 20% of cases, and might present as a mass in the flank or pain after drinking. It is thought to result from abnormal smooth muscle organization at the ureteropelvic junction. It can be accompanied by renal agenesis of the opposite kidney; the reason for this is unknown. As a result of the back pressure from the obstruction, the pelvic-alyceal system dilates. If the pressure is transmitted to the kidneys, the renal tissue atrophies. If bilateral, renal failure can result.

Diverticula

Diverticula are outpouchings of the ureteral wall; they are usually congenital. They are very common and create sites for the stasis of urine. This increases the risk of urine infection because the continuous flow of urine through the urinary tract is a protective mechanism against infection. Acquired diverticula can develop if the pressure in the ureters increases (e.g. because of obstruction).

Hydroureter and megaloureter

Congenital hydroureters develop if there are neuromuscular defects in the wall of the ureter. They are sometimes associated with other congenital malformations in the genitourinary tract. There is dilatation, elongation and frequently tortuosity of the ureters. Acquired hydroureters develop in adults during pregnancy and lower urinary tract obstruction, where a persistently raised pressure within the bladder impairs ureter emptying. A ureter so dilated that transport of urine by peristalsis is compromised is known as a megaloureter.

Bladder abnormalities

Diverticula

These are sac-like outpouchings through a weak point in the bladder wall. They can be either:

- Congenital: these develop in localized areas of defective muscle within the wall or because of urinary tract obstruction in fetal development. They are usually solitary lesions, most commonly occurring close to the ureterovesical junction.
- Acquired: these usually develop much later in life as a result of chronic urethral obstruction (e.g. prostatic hypertrophy). They are clinically significant and, characteristically, occur as multiple lesions.

In both cases, urine stasis increases the risk of bladder infection, leading to vesicoureteric reflux and eventual stone formation.

Exstrophy

Exstrophy of the bladder is a serious condition affecting the anterior wall of the bladder and anterior abdominal wall. It presents in infancy and is more common in males. The anterior wall of the bladder fails to develop, so the posterior wall lies exposed on the lower abdominal wall, causing squamous metaplasia of the mucosa. The mucosa is at high risk of infection. This disorder can vary in severity and can be associated with urethral and symphysis pubis defects. In the male there is epispadias, and in females a split clitoris. Surgical correction allows long-term survival of these infants. Despite treatment, there is an increased risk of adenocarcinoma of the bladder later in life, because of bladder extrusion.

Urethral abnormalities

Hypospadias

This is a spectrum of congenital abnormalities affecting 1 in 400 male infants. The urethra opens on the ventral surface of the penis, usually adjacent to the glans penis, but can open on the penile shaft or perineum. There is a ventral curvature to the penile shaft with a hooded prepuce. Surgical correction is usually carried out before the age of 2 years to allow micturition with a straight stream.

Epispadias

The urethra opens on the dorsal surface of the penis. As with hypospadias, surgical correction is usually carried out before the age of 2 years to allow micturition with a straight stream.

Urethral valves

Obstruction to urine flow can occur at the level of the posterior urethra in a boy due to the presence of mucosal folds or a membrane extending across the urethra (posterior urethral valve). The patient presents in early infancy with distended bladder, dribbling, vomiting and failure to thrive. As a result of obstruction to urinary flow, male fetuses can have:

- Poor renal growth with reflux and dilated upper urinary tracts
- Progressive bilateral hydronephrosis
- Oligohydramnios (reduced volume of amniotic fluid).

Intrauterine intervention has no proven benefit and an early delivery is performed only if there are signs of rapidly progressing renal damage. Postnatal management includes:

- Prophylactic antibiotics from birth to prevent urinary tract infections (UTI)
- Ultrasound scans at birth and a few weeks later to assess the effect of the obstruction.

Surgical treatment is required in all cases. Any male child born with bilateral hydronephrosis must be investigated to exclude a posterior urethral valve.

URINARY TRACT OBSTRUCTION AND UROLITHIASIS

Urinary tract obstruction

Obstruction in the urinary tract can occur at any level. It can be unilateral or bilateral, complete or incomplete, and of gradual or acute onset. It increases the risk of UTI, reflux and stone formation. If prolonged or unrelieved, obstruction can cause functional renal impairment and permanent renal atrophy. Imaging techniques involved in the diagnosis of urinary tract obstruction and its location (see Chapter 8) are as follows:

- Computed tomography (CT) or magnetic resonance imaging (MRI): these provide good anatomical definition and can identify the cause and level of obstruction. They have become the imaging modality of choice in centres where they are readily available.
- Ultrasound: this can readily identify dilatation of the urinary tract and avoids exposure to ionizing radiation so can be used repetitively and in children.
- DTPA (diethylenetriamine penta-acetic acid) renography: this is used to confirm whether dilatation of the renal tract is the result of functional obstruction.
- Intravenous urography (IVU): this can highlight the level and cause of obstruction (now used less commonly and should be avoided in patients with impaired renal function).

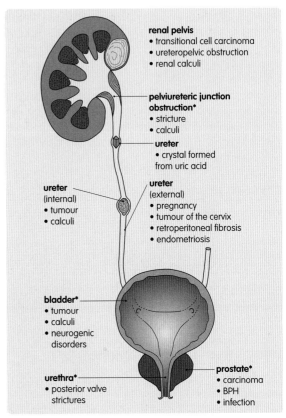

Fig. 5.11 Sites of obstruction in the urinary tract.* The most common sites of obstruction. BPH, benign prostatic hyperplasia.

- Retrograde pyelography: this can be necessary to define the cause of obstruction in some cases.

Careful imaging of the renal tract is essential to determine the site and cause of obstruction (see Chapter 8).

Causes of urinary obstruction

Figure 5.11 shows the sites of obstruction in the urinary tract. Obstruction is caused by a congenital defect or, more commonly, by a structural lesion.

Congenital abnormalities
These include the following neuromuscular defects:

- Urethral valves and strictures
- Meatal strictures
- Bladder neck obstruction
- Ureteropelvic obstruction or stenosis.

Mechanical obstruction of the meatus and urethra occurs only in boys. Severe vesicoureteric reflux eventually results in upper renal tract dilatation without obstruction.

Tumours

Tumours can cause obstruction in two ways:

1. Internal: tumours within the urinary tract wall or lumen (e.g. bladder carcinoma). These occupy the urinary tract lumen, causing direct obstruction.
2. External: pressure from rectal or prostate tumours or from gynaecological malignancies narrows the urinary tract lumen, causing indirect obstruction.

Calculi (urolithiasis)

Stones in the urinary tract can cause urinary obstruction.

Pregnancy

The high levels of progesterone in pregnancy relax smooth muscle fibres in the renal pelvis and ureters and cause a dysfunctional obstruction. There might also be external compression from the pressure of the enlarging fetus on the ureters.

Hyperplastic lesions

The most common hyperplastic lesion causing urinary obstruction is benign prostatic hypertrophy (BPH).

Inflammation

Any inflammation in the lower urinary tract will cause an obstruction (e.g. urethritis, ureteritis, prostatitis, retroperitoneal fibrosis). Obstruction resolves with the treatment of the inflammation.

Neurogenic disorders

These result from:

- Congenital anomalies affecting the spinal cord (e.g. spina bifida).
- External pressure on the cord or lumbar nerve roots (e.g. meningioma, lumbar disc prolapse).
- Trauma to the spinal cord.

Hydronephrosis

This is dilatation of the renal pelvis and calyces due to obstruction at any point in the urinary tract causing increased pressure above the blockage. It can be:

- Unilateral: caused by an upper urinary tract obstruction. This is detected late because renal function is maintained by the other kidney. Thus, the affected kidney can be severely impaired by the time obstruction is detected.
- Bilateral: because of obstruction in the lower urinary tract. Renal failure develops earlier and prompt intervention is required to prevent chronic renal failure.

Progressive atrophy of the kidney develops as the back pressure from the obstruction is transmitted to the distal parts of the nephron. The glomerular filtration rate (GFR) declines and, if the obstruction is bilateral, the patient goes into renal failure. Progressive damage to the renal structures results in flattening of the calyces with gradual thinning of the renal parenchyma, eventually leaving a cystic, thin-walled, fibrous sac with no functional capacity.

- Obstruction at the pyeloureteral junction: hydronephrosis.
- Obstruction of the ureter: hydroureter, eventually developing hydronephrosis.
- Obstruction of the bladder neck/urethra: bladder distension with hypertrophy, eventually leading to hydroureter and thus hydronephrosis. If bilateral, renal failure develops earlier.

Presentation of urinary obstruction

This depends on the site and cause of the obstruction:

- An acute complete obstruction in the ureters (e.g. due to a stone) causes severe renal colic. If bilateral, the patient is at risk of acute renal failure
- Gradual obstruction (e.g. prostatic hypertrophy) causes bladder distension with hesitancy, terminal dribbling, poor urine flow and a sense of incomplete voiding
- A unilateral and partial obstruction causing a hydroureter or hydronephrosis might not be apparent for many years because the unaffected kidney maintains adequate renal function
- A bilateral and partial obstruction presents with nocturia and polyuria caused by tubular cell dysfunction with an inability to concentrate urine. Other chronic manifestations include renal stones, salt wasting, distal renal tubular acidosis and hypertension. If undiagnosed, the patient develops chronic renal failure
- A bilateral and complete obstruction presents as anuria or oliguria and must be treated urgently. Following removal of the obstruction, there may be a postobstructive diuresis which can result in

dehydration if not managed appropriately. Any general malaise or fever might be a sign of superimposed infection.

In all cases, the prompt and effective relief of the obstruction is essential. Depending on the site this may require a urinary catheter, urinary stent or a nephrostomy (to allow renal function to improve), followed by surgical intervention.

- Sudden and complete obstruction causes a significant fall in GFR, resulting in acute renal failure.
- Partial or chronic obstruction does not affect the GFR, so renal function is impaired gradually.

Urolithiasis (urinary calculi)

Incidence and risk factors

Urinary calculi affect 1–5% of the population and are more common in men. They are formed by precipitation of urinary components along with a small core of organic material, and form anywhere along the urinary tract, most commonly in the renal pelvis. Calculi vary in size and number. Risk factors for stone formation include:

- Increased solute in the urine as a result of high plasma levels (e.g. calcium and urate) or abnormal tubular function (e.g. calcium and cysteine)
- Absence of inhibiting substances (e.g. citrate and phosphate)
- Acidic urinary pH, which reduces solubility of a substance in the urine
- Urinary stasis or obstruction.

Occasionally, a calculus can grow to take up the shape of the renal pelvis and branch into calyces (staghorn calculus). Stone formation is initiated by a core of mucoproteins or urates (nucleation); as more components deposit on the core, the stone gradually increases in size (aggregation). Figure 5.12 lists the different types of stone and their frequency.

Fig. 5.12 Different types of renal stone and their frequency

Type	Frequency (%)

calcium-containing stones:
   calcium oxalate
   calcium phosphate
	
	60–70
	10–15

complex triple stones (magnesium, aluminium, phosphate)	15
uric acid stones	5
cysteine stones	1–2

Presentation

The clinical presentation includes:

- Renal colic due to the increase in peristalsis in the ureters in response to the passage of small stones along the ureter
- A continuous dull ache in the loins due to kidney stones
- Strangury: the urge to pass something that will not pass (bladder stone)
- Recurrent and untreatable UTIs, haematuria or renal failure
- Asymptomatic.

Treatment

Management involves adequate analgesia and a high fluid intake. Stones less than 0.5 cm in diameter usually pass spontaneously; larger stones might require surgical intervention. Treatment options include:

- Percutaneous surgery: endoscopic removal of the stone
- Open surgical removal
- Extracorporeal lithotripsy: shock waves are used to fragment the calculi into small pieces which will then pass out in the urine.

Prevention of renal stones involves:

- A high fluid intake to produce a dilute urine
- Treatment for an underlying metabolic abnormality
- Combination of the above.

INFLAMMATION OF THE URINARY TRACT

Ureteritis

This is inflammation of the ureter and can occur in UTI. Persistent or recurrent infection leads to chronic inflammation, which has two reaction patterns:

1. Ureteritis folliculitis: lymphocytic aggregation under the epithelium causes elevation of the mucosal surface with a fine granular appearance.
2. Ureteritis cystica: multiple small cysts (1–5 mm) develop from fibrosed clumps of epithelial cells on the surface of the ureteric mucosa. They are thin walled with clear fluid, and project into the lumen.

Cystitis

This is inflammation of the urinary bladder and is common in UTI. It can be acute or chronic. The aetiology and predisposing factors were discussed with UTI (see p. 78). The pathogens that cause cystitis are:

- Most common: *Escherichia coli* and *Proteus* species, followed by *Enterobacter*
- *Candida albicans* in patients on long-term antibiotics
- *Cryptococcus* species in immunosuppressed patients
- *Schistosoma* species, particularly in Middle Eastern countries
- *Mycobacterium tuberculosis*: tuberculous cystitis usually suggests tuberculosis in the upper urinary tract.

Sterile cystitis can be caused by radiation damage, drugs and instrumentation. Ascending infection following cystitis can cause pyelonephritis.

> Cystitis is inflammation of the urinary bladder, common in UTI. It can be acute or chronic, and the most serious complication is pyelonephritis.

Acute cystitis

In acute cystitis the mucosa becomes hyperaemic, often producing an exudate. There are various forms:

- Haemorrhagic cystitis: occurs if the hyperaemia becomes excessive, resulting in bleeding
- Exudative cystitis: yellow areas of fibrinous exudate develop on the mucosa
- Suppurative cystitis: large quantities of exudate accumulate
- Ulcerative cystitis: large areas of ulceration occur in the bladder mucosa
- Gangrenous cystitis: as a result of ischaemia, which results in areas of black necrotic bladder mucosa.

Chronic cystitis

This results from recurrent or persistent infection of the bladder. Chronic infection leads to fibrous thickening, so the bladder wall is less distensible. This affects the ability of the bladder to store urine and contract during micturition.

Other types of cystitis

Interstitial cystitis

This type of cystitis is often associated with systemic lupus erythematosus, so is thought to be an auto-immune condition. As with all autoimmune conditions, it has a much higher incidence in women than in men. It can also result from recurrent and persistent infection that leads to fibrosis of all the layers of the bladder wall. There is often localized ulceration of the mucosa.

Malakoplakia vesicae

This is a very rare form of chronic bacterial cystitis, but it is important because it can mimic a tumour. Raised mucosal plaques of inflammation cells develop on the bladder and ureteric mucosa. These plaques are inflammatory, soft, yellow, 3–5 cm in diameter and are prone to ulceration. On histological examination the plaques are found to contain foamy macrophages with a granular cytoplasm containing Michaelis–Gutmann bodies and chronic inflammatory cells. Malakoplakia is more common in renal transplant patients.

Presentation and treatment

The classic symptoms of all types of cystitis are:

- Urgency and frequency of micturition
- Dysuria
- Lower abdominal pain and tenderness.

There might be associated systemic signs of fever, general malaise and rigours.

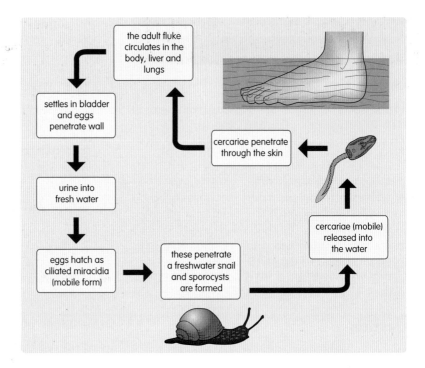

Fig. 5.13 Infestation with
S. haematobium.

Treatment of cystitis involves a 3–5-day course of antibiotics with a high fluid intake. Recurrent infection should always be investigated.

Schistosomiasis (bilharzia)

Schistosomiasis is the most common helminth infection worldwide, although it is rare in the UK. It is endemic in the Middle East, Africa, the Far East and in parts of South America. The pathogen is a blood fluke (*Schistosoma haematobium*). Humans are infected via freshwater snails, which contain cercariae – parasites in the cercarial phase of development. The schistosomes penetrate intact skin to enter the venous system, and thus migrate to the liver and bladder. They settle in the bladder to lay eggs causing chronic irritation of the transitional cells of the bladder. The eggs are excreted into local water supplies and transmitted through freshwater snails (Fig. 5.13).

People infected with cercariae can present with an itchy papular rash accompanied by myalgia, abdominal pain and headache. The most common presentation of infection with *S. haematobium* is recurrent haematuria. Eventually, urinary tract obstruction, bladder calcification (predisposing to squamous carcinoma) and renal failure occur.

Diagnosis involves:

- Urine sample to detect the eggs in the urine.
- Enzyme-linked immunosorbent assay (ELISA) to detect a response to infection.

Treatment is with praziquantel given once daily.

Metaplasia associated with bladder exstrophy, chronic bladder inflammation and schistosomiasis is a premalignant condition.

Urethral inflammation

The most common pathogens are *E. coli* and *Proteus* species. Ascending infection including cystitis, ureteritis and pyelitis can result.

Acute inflammation of the urethra occurs from infection with a sexually transmitted disease (e.g. *Neisseria gonorrhoeae* or *Chlamydia trachomatis*) (see *Crash Course: Endocrine and Reproductive System* for further details). Urethritis is seen with conjunctivitis and arthritis in Reiter's disease.

NEOPLASTIC DISEASE OF THE URINARY TRACT

Tumours of the ureters

These are rare.

Benign tumours of the ureter

These originate from blood vessels, lymphatics and smooth muscle. A fibroepithelial polyp is a small mass that projects into the lumen. It consists of a clump of vascular connective tissue beneath the ureteric mucosa.

Malignant tumours of the ureters

Primary malignancies are rare and metastatic disease is relatively more common in the ureters. Malignant tumours arise from the transitional epithelium lining the ureters and most of the urinary tract. They are usually asymptomatic for many years and are found in 60–70-year-olds. They eventually present as a partial and unilateral obstruction as the ureteric lumen becomes occluded. They often occur in association with multiple tumours of the bladder and renal pelvis (synchronous tumours of the uroepithelium).

Tumours of the bladder

Metaplasia

The transitional cell lining (urothelium) of the bladder can undergo metaplastic changes during any period of infection or inflammation as a result of stones, drugs and radiation. There are three types of metaplasia:

1. Squamous metaplasia: this occurs in areas of long-term chronic inflammation in bladder exstrophy, bladder calculi, and schistosomiasis. It is a risk factor for squamous cell carcinoma.
2. Intestinal or glandular metaplasia: this is associated with chronic cystitis and leads to the formation of slit-like glands of columnar epithelium.
3. Nephrogenic metaplasia (rare): this is associated with chronic infections. The urothelium is transformed to cuboidal epithelium, and must be differentiated from adenocarcinoma.

Benign tumours of the bladder

These are rare, accounting for 2–3% of bladder epithelial tumours. Transitional cell papilloma can be the first stage (grade I) of transitional cell carcinoma. These papillomas are often multiple and are found all over the mucosal lining. They are small projections (0.5–2.0 cm in length) with uniform cellular structure. They attach to the mucosa by a small stalk with a fibrovascular core covered in urothelium.

The other benign lesions are inverted papillomas. These consist of solitary nodules in the mucosa and measure 1–3 cm in diameter.

Transitional cell carcinomas

These are malignant tumours that arise from the transitional cell epithelium that lines the bladder. They account for over 90% of bladder epithelial cell tumours, and the number of cases is increasing. They are uncommon under 50 years of age and more commonly affect males (4 males:1 female).

> The most common urinary tract malignancy is transitional cell carcinoma and the most common site is the bladder. In countries where schistosomiasis is endemic, squamous cell carcinoma of the bladder is common.

Presentation

The most common presentation of any tumour of the bladder is painless haematuria. This is often accompanied by symptoms of a UTI (i.e. dysuria, frequency and urgency). Symptoms can also be caused by local invasion of the tumour causing ureteric obstruction. Risk factors include:

- Smoking
- Exposure to chemicals in the rubber industry (e.g. naphthylamine and benzidine)
- Analgesic misuse.

Pathology

There are two main types of transitional cell tumour (Fig. 5.14):

1. Papillary tumour (70%): this is a wart-like lesion covered in a thick layer of urothelium

branching off a stalk that attaches it to the mucosa (as described above).

2. Sessile (flat) tumour: these are plaques of thickened mucosa with a well-defined border.

Both these types of tumour can be in situ or invasive:

- In situ carcinomas: these are flat lesions that are confined to the mucosa of the upper urinary tract or bladder. They are the precursors of the invasive tumours.
- Invasive tumours: these infiltrate the basement membrane of the bladder mucosa and the lamina propria and can penetrate adjacent structures once through the mucosal wall.

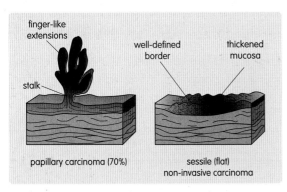

Fig. 5.14 Papillary and sessile transitional cell tumours.

Transitional cell carcinomas can be graded according to the degree of cellular abnormalities on histological examination:

- Grade I: there is an increase in the number of well-differentiated epithelial cell layers (>7) and there is some cell atypia.
- Grade II: there is an increase in cell layers (>10) and there is a large variation in cell size and in nucleus shape and size (i.e. moderately well differentiated).
- Grade III: the cells have no resemblance to their cells of origin (poorly differentiated), with breakdown of connections between the cells causing them to fragment.

As tumour growth progresses, the relatively benign, well-differentiated papillary growths (grade I) can eventually form solid, plaque-like anaplastic tumours (grade III). Grade III tumours are often ulcerated and have penetrated through the bladder muscle wall. They are associated with the worst prognosis. Carcinomas with over 5% squamous or glandular metaplasia are called mixed tumours.

The TNM system is used for the staging of transitional cell tumours, i.e. to assess the extent of spread (Fig. 5.15). This has been correlated to grade. Tumour spread can be:

- Local: invasion into the bladder wall and to adjacent pelvic structures

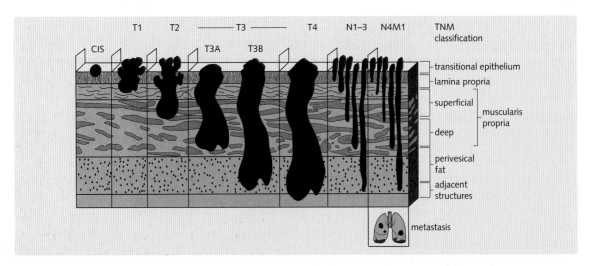

Fig. 5.15 TNM staging system for transitional cell carcinoma of bladder. T staging describes tumour invasion of the tissue layers. N staging describes the degree of spread to the lymph nodes: 1, local nodes; 2, distant nodes below the diaphragm; 3, distant nodes on both sides of the diaphragm. M staging describes the presence or absence of metastases: 0, none; 1, present. CIS, carcinoma in situ (from Bahnson RR 1994 Management of urologic disorders. Mosby Year Book).

- Distant: lymphatic spread to the periaortic lymph nodes or haematological metastases to the liver and lungs.

Investigation via cystoscopy and biopsy allows histological examination, which confirms whether there is muscle involvement. The distinction between the lamina propria invasion and submucosal invasion is correlated with the prognosis.

Most of the tumours are situated on the posterior and lateral walls of the bladder, and are often multiple. This suggests that the entire epithelium is unstable as a result of the constant exposure to the carcinogens being excreted in urine.

Diagnosis, treatment and prognosis

Diagnosis is made by cytological examination of the urine to check for the presence of malignant cells and by cystoscopy of the lower urinary tract.

Treatment depends on the stage and histological grade of the tumour:

- T1 tumours: tumour resection using diathermy (via cystoscopy) with close follow-up
- T2/3 tumours: radiotherapy and cystectomy
- T4 tumours: palliative radiotherapy.

Intravesicular chemotherapy, and more recently, intravesicular BCG (bacille Calmette Guérin) treatment have been shown to be effective in treating bladder cancer.

The average 5-year survival rate is 80% if the bladder wall is not involved and 5% if there is local invasion on presentation. Patients with fixed tumours and metastases have a median survival of 1 year.

Squamous cell carcinoma

These usually arise in areas of squamous metaplasia of the bladder mucosa and account for <10% of bladder carcinomas. Risk factors include bladder exstrophy, chronic inflammation, calculi and schistosomiasis, which cause chronic irritation to the transitional cells of the bladder, leading to squamous metaplasia. This becomes dysplastic, resulting in carcinoma in situ, which can progress to invasive squamous cell carcinoma.

The tumours are solid, ulcerative, invasive and fungating masses, and are often very extensive on discovery. Their prognosis is worse than that of transitional cell carcinoma.

Adenocarcinoma

This is rare in the bladder and usually occurs in the urachal remnants, at the apex of the bladder. Histological examination shows metaplasia of the transitional epithelium or cystitis cystica.

The most common site for bladder tumours to develop is the posterior and lateral walls (70%) followed by the trigone and bladder neck (20%).

DISORDERS OF THE PROSTATE

Prostatitis

There are three subgroups of inflammation of the prostate.

Acute prostatitis

The main pathogens are *E. coli*, *Proteus* and *Staphylococcus* species, and sexually transmitted pathogens including *C. trachomatis* and *Neisseria gonorrhoeae*. Inflammation can be focal or diffuse. Infection is usually spread from an acute infection in the urethra or bladder because of:

- Intraprostatic reflux of urine
- Intraprostatic catheterization
- Surgical manipulation of the urethra (e.g. cystoscopy).

Occasionally, acute prostatitis is caused by a blood-borne infection.

On histological examination there is an acute inflammatory infiltrate of neutrophils and damaged cells, often resulting in abscess formation.

Patients present with:

- General symptoms: malaise, rigours and fever.
- Local symptoms: difficulty in passing urine, dysuria and perineal tenderness.

Rectal examination reveals a soft, tender and enlarged prostate. Diagnosis is based on the clinical features and a positive urine culture.

Chronic prostatitis

This results from inadequately treated acute infection. This can occur because some antibiotics cannot penetrate the prostate effectively. There is often a history of recurrent prostatic and urinary tract infections. Causative pathogens are the same as for acute prostatic infection.

Patients present with dysuria and low back and perineal pain, with no preceding acute phase. Some patients are asymptomatic.

Chronic prostatitis is difficult to diagnose and treat. Diagnosis is confirmed by:

- Histological examination showing neutrophils, plasma cells and lymphocytes
- A positive culture from a sample of prostatic secretion.

Tuberculosis is a cause of chronic infection and can affect the kidneys or epididymis. Histological examination reveals focal areas of caseation and giant cell infiltrates.

Chronic non-bacterial prostatitis

This is the most common type of prostatitis and results in enlargement of the prostate, which can obstruct the urethra. The usual pathogen is *C. trachomatis* so, typically, sexually active men are affected. Often there is no history of recurrent UTIs.

Presentation is similar to that of chronic prostatitis and histological examination shows fibrosis as a result of chronic inflammation.

Diagnosis is confirmed by the presence of 15 white blood cells per high power field (this indicates inflammation) and repeated negative bacterial cultures (excludes infection).

Benign prostatic hypertrophy

Incidence

BPH is detectable to some extent in nearly all men over the age of 60. It is a non-neoplastic enlargement of the prostate gland, which can eventually lead to bladder outflow obstruction. The cause is unknown, but might be related to levels of male sex hormones (testosterone).

Presentation

Symptoms develop as the enlarging gland compresses the prostatic urethra and the periurethral glands (known as the median lobe) swell, affecting the bladder sphincter mechanism. Men present with 'prostatism', a triad of:

- Difficulty or hesitancy in starting to urinate
- A poor stream
- Dribbling postmicturition, frequency and nocturia
  Examination must include:
- Abdominal examination for an enlarged palpable bladder
- Digital rectal examination for the prostate, which is firm, smooth and rubbery.

Untreated BPH can present with acute urinary retention, which is accompanied by a distended and tender bladder and a desperate urge to pass urine. Alternatively, the patient might have progressive bladder distension, leading to chronic painless retention and overflow incontinence. If undetected, BPH can lead to bilateral upper tract obstruction and renal impairment, with the patient presenting in chronic renal failure (see Chapter 6).

Enlarging of the prostate gland in BPH presents with:

- Hesitancy in starting urination
- Poor stream
- Dribbling postmicturition
- Frequency
- Nocturia.

Pathology

There is hyperplasia of both the lateral lobes and the median lobes (these lie behind the urethra), leading to compression of the urethra and therefore bladder outflow obstruction. Within the prostate there are solid nodules of fibromuscular material and cystic regions. Histological examination shows hyperplasia of the:

- Stroma (smooth muscle and fibrous tissue)
- Glands, often with areas of infarction and necrosis.

Complications

The complications of BPH develop from prolonged obstruction to urine flow. There is compensatory hypertrophy of the bladder as a result of the high pressures that develop within the bladder (Fig. 5.16).

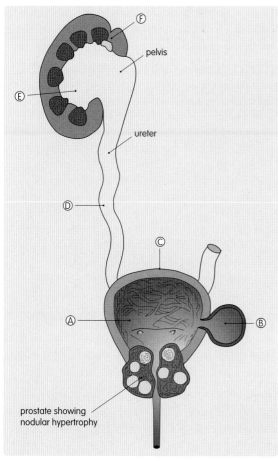

pelvis

ureter

prostate showing
nodular hypertrophy

Fig. 5.16 Complications of benign prostatic hypertrophy. (A) Bands of thickened smooth muscle fibres cause trabeculation of the bladder wall. (B) Diverticula can develop on the external surface of the bladder. (C) Dilatation of the bladder once the muscle becomes hypotonic. (D) Formation of hydroureters resulting in the reflux of urine up to the renal pelvis. (E) Bilateral hydronephrosis. (F) Kidney infection, stones, calculi and renal failure.

Treatment

- Medical treatment: symptoms can be improved with α-blockers (which relax smooth muscle at the bladder neck, thus improving urinary flow rate) and antiandrogens such as finasteride. Finasteride is a 5α-reductase inhibitor that prevents the conversion of testosterone to the more potent androgen dihydrotestosterone. Dihydrotestosterone promotes growth and enlargement of the prostate; inhibition of its production causes gradual reduction in prostate volume, thereby improving urinary flow rate and obstructive symptoms.

- Surgical treatment: transurethral resection of the prostate (TURP) is quick and safe with low mortality and a good success rate.

Carcinoma of the prostate

Incidence and risk factors

Prostate cancer is the third most common cancer in men (after cancer of the lung and stomach), accounting for 8% of all cancers in men. It is a disease of elderly men, occurring in 1 in 10 men of 70 years of age. It is rare under 55 years of age and has a strong hereditary component.

The cause is unknown, but there is a link between androgenic hormones and tumour growth. The lesions are most commonly found in the periphery of the posterior part of the prostate compared with the more central and lateral location of BPH – these areas have different embryological origins and often both conditions coexist.

Presentation

Patients present with symptoms of UTI, prostatism or metastatic disease in the bone (usually the spine) causing bone pain. Carcinoma can be found coincidentally in autopsies of elderly men who were asymptomatic. About 25% of patients have symptoms of metastatic disease on presentation (anaemia, ureteric obstruction or bone pain that is worse at night). Increasingly carcinoma of the prostate is discovered following investigation of elevated prostate-specific antigen (PSA) in otherwise asymptomatic men. The value of early diagnosis in long-term outcome is currently unclear.

Pathology

The tumours range from well-differentiated single nodules to anaplastic and diffuse involvement of all lobes of the gland. The Gleason classification is used to grade the tumours on histological appearance. Grade 1 is a well-differentiated tumour composed of uniform tumour cells whereas grade 5 is an anaplastic diffuse tumour with cells showing great variation in their structure and a high mitotic rate.

As for transitional cell carcinoma of the bladder, stage is determined by the TNM system:

- T_1: unsuspected impalpable tumour
- T_2: the tumour is confined to the prostate
- T_3: there is local extension of the tumour beyond the prostatic capsule

- T_4: the tumour has fixed to other local structures.

Tumour spread can be by:

- Local invasion of adjacent structures, including the bladder and ureters
- Lymphatic spread to the iliac and periaortic nodes
- Haematogenous spread to the bones of the spine and pelvis and occasionally to the lungs and liver.

Diagnosis

- Digital rectal examination: hard and irregular prostate.
- Ultrasound: used to define a prostatic mass.
- PSA level in the blood: this increases in prostate cancer, but a normal result does not exclude the presence of cancer.
- Serum prostatic acid phosphatase: this also increases, especially if there are metastases.
- Biopsy of the prostate (using a transrectal approach under ultrasound guidance (TRUS)) is required to provide a histological diagnosis.
- Radiographs and bone scans: used to stage the tumour. Osteosclerotic lesions on radiographs and increased isotope uptake on bone scans are seen if there is metastatic spread (see Chapter 8).

Treatment and prognosis

Treatment options include surgery, hormone therapy and radiotherapy. Before treatment is started, a histological diagnosis of prostatic carcinoma is required. Treatment depends on the stage of the tumour:

- T1/T2 staged tumours: radical surgical resection of the prostate (prostatectomy) may be curative. TURP might also be required in advanced metastatic disease to relieve the symptoms of urethral obstruction.
- Local radiotherapy can be used if the patient is unfit for surgery, and to treat local or distant spread of the tumour. It can provide useful palliation for bony metastases.
- Advanced tumours: hormonal manipulation is beneficial since testosterone promotes tumour growth. Thus, removal of both testes (orchidectomy) blocking the source of testosterone, will cause the tumour to shrink, although this is rarely used now. Luteinizing-hormone-releasing hormone (LHRH) analogues (e.g. buserelin) prevent testosterone release are equally effective and are increasingly used. Antiandrogens such as cyproterone acetate are also used to block testosterone action.

Prognosis depends on stage. The 5-year survival rate for T1 tumours is 75–90%. However, the 5-year survival falls to 30–45% if there is local or metastatic spread.

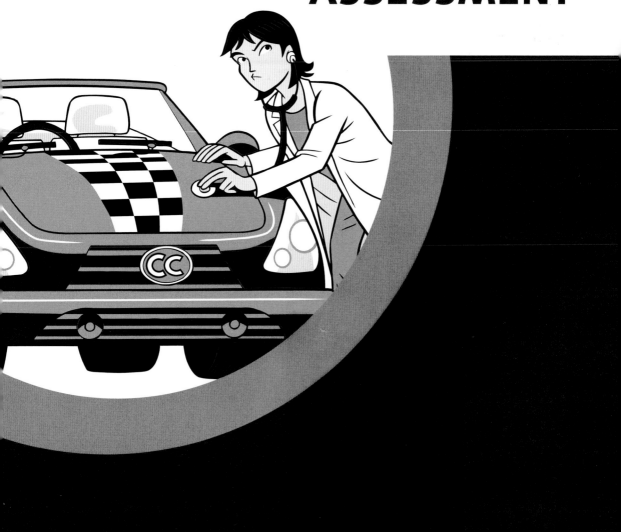

CLINICAL ASSESSMENT

Common presentations of renal disease

Objectives

By the end of the chapter you should be able to:

- Explain the difference between frequency and urgency
- Interpret urinalysis
- Explain what pseudohyponatraemia is and how it is diagnosed
- Describe the effect of tissue necrosis on total body K^+, and why this must be corrected urgently
- Classify the causes of acute renal failure
- Understand how to identify and manage chronic kidney disease
- Name and define five types of incontinence, and discuss the risk factors for developing incontinence
- Outline the risk factors for and common causes of urinary tract infections
- Define the nephrotic syndrome and list common primary and secondary causes
- Outline the tests required to identify chlamydia in a patient presenting with urethral discharge
- List the three principles of treating patients with sexually transmitted infections.

Introduction

Renal disease can present in numerous ways. In this chapter each presentation will be dealt with individually. Many of these, however, are non-specific and renal disease can be asymptomatic until a very late stage. It is therefore essential to have a systematic approach to diagnosis which should include:

- Blood pressure measurement
- Urinalysis (mid-stream urine).

BLOOD AND URINE ABNORMALITIES

Haematuria

Blood in the urine can be:

- Microscopic: blood is visible only under a microscope or on dipstick analysis
- Macroscopic ('frank' haematuria): blood is visible with the naked eye (>5 red blood cells per high-power field).

The degree of haematuria does not always reflect the severity of the underlying disorder.

Causes

Causes of haematuria are:

- Renal causes: glomerular disease such as primary glomerulonephritis (e.g. IgA nephropathy), disorders secondary to systemic illness (e.g. vasculitis, systemic lupus erythematosus (SLE)), carcinoma (both renal and transitional cell), trauma, cystic disease, emboli.
- Extrarenal causes: urinary tract infection (UTI)*, ureteral calculi*, prostatic hypertrophy*, carcinoma of the bladder*, renal stone*, trauma, urethritis, catheterization, post-cyclophosphamide.
- Systemic causes: coagulation disorders, sickle-cell trait or disease.
- Others: anticoagulant drugs.

(*Indicates the most common causes.)

Dipsticks detect haemoglobin (not red blood cells) and will give positive results if there is intra-vascular haemolysis, since haemoglobin is filtered freely by glomeruli (haemoglobinuria). This can occur physiologically, after heavy exercise, during pregnancy or with prosthetic heart valves. If haemolysis is severe (i.e. in haemolytic crisis), the urine can become red.

Fig. 6.1 Common sites of lesions causing haematuria. BPH, benign prostatic hypertrophy.

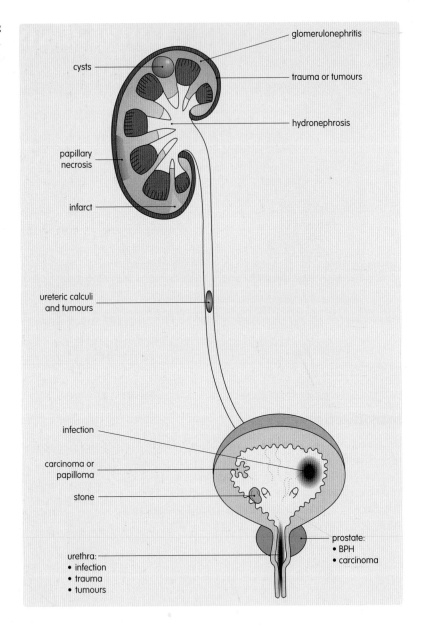

Other conditions can cause a red-brown discoloration of the urine that can be confused with haematuria (e.g. porphyria, myoglobinuria, ingestion of some foods (beetroot) or drugs (phenolphthalein)).

Diagnostic approach

Figure 6.1 shows the common sites of lesions causing haematuria. The investigative approach for haematuria is shown in Figure 6.2. A flow chart summarizing further investigation of haematuria if the intravenous pyelogram (IVP) or ultrasound result is abnormal is given in Figure 6.3. The significance of urinalysis is summarized in Figure 6.4.

Proteinuria

Proteinuria is the presence of excess protein in the urine. It is usually assessed using a dipstick, which detects protein levels above 300 mg/L. 'Microalbuminuria' is the presence of excess urinary albumin but in amounts insufficient to cause a positive dipstick analysis. Proteinuria is best measured as the protein concentration on a 'spot' (early morning) urine sample corrected for urine

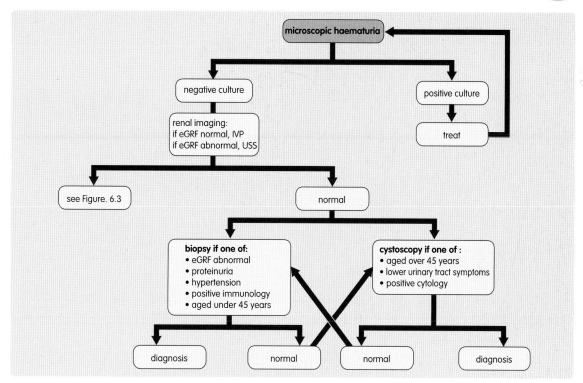

Fig. 6.2 Investigation of haematuria. eGRF, estimated glomerular filtration rate; IVP, intravenous pyelography; USS, ultrasound scan.

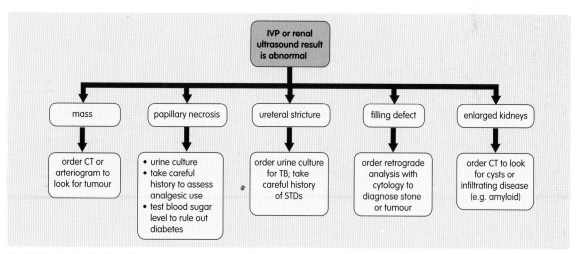

Fig. 6.3 Further investigation of haematuria when the IVP or ultrasound result is abnormal. CT, computed tomography; IVP, intravenous pyelography; STD, sexually transmitted disease; TB, tuberculosis (from Green HL 1996 Clinical medicine, 2nd edn. Mosby Year Book).

creatinine concentration (protein to creatinine ratio or albumin to creatinine ratio). It may also be quantified on 24-h urine collections to give the amount excreted in 24 h but this is difficult to perform accurately. The amount of protein excreted can vary through the day and may increase with up-right posture (orthostatic proteinuria). Urine usually contains <20 mg/L of albumin and <200 mg/day of protein (exact values vary from laboratory to laboratory according to methods used to measure protein). Proteinuria is seen in diabetic nephropathy. As well as being a risk factor for progressive chronic

121

Fig. 6.4 Urine analysis – findings and their interpretations

Findings	Possible diagnoses
clots in urine	carcinoma of the bladder or kidney clot colic is also a feature of IgA nephropathy
albuminuria and haematuria red blood cell casts	intrinsic renal disease glomerulonephritis – red cell casts are pathognomic of active glomerular bleeding (e.g. IgA, nephropathy, vasculitis)
haematuria, pyuria and white blood cell casts	renal tubulointerstitial disease – this is a non-specific diagnosis (i.e. pyelonephritis)
dysmorphic red cells	glomerular bleeding (i.e. glomerulonephritis)

kidney disease (CKD), proteinuria is also associated with increased cardiovascular risk in hypertension and ischaemic heart disease.

Causes

Causes of proteinuria are summarized, together with relevant investigations, in Figure 6.5.

Nephrotic syndrome

This is characterized by proteinuria (usually >3 g/day), sufficient to cause a decrease in serum albumin (hypoalbuminaemia) and hence oedema. It is associated with a secondary increase in cholesterol (hypercholesterolaemia). Primary nephrotic syndrome results from diseases arising in the glomerulus. These include:

- Commonly, minimal change glomerulonephritis, membranous glomerulonephritis,

Fig. 6.5 Causes and investigation of proteinuria

Cause	Investigation
urinary tract infection	mid-stream urine sample and culture
diabetic nephropathy	blood glucose levels (glucose tolerance test) examination for other diabetic complications
glomerulonephritis	biopsy (for histological diagnosis) blood pressure
nephrotic syndrome	cholesterol levels, oedema
congestive cardiac failure	clinical signs, blood pressure
hypertension	regular blood pressure measurements renal biopsy
myeloma	full blood count serum and urine protein electrophoresis bone marrow biopsy
amyloid	biopsy and Congo red staining look for associated splenomegaly
pregnancy	hCG pregnancy test
pyrexia	core temperature measurement at regular intervals
exercise	urine sample on waking to be repeated following exercise
postural proteinuria (rare if >30 years old)	urine sample on waking repeated at mid-day
vaginal mucus contaminant	repeat urine sample, with sterile technique

Note: hCG, human chorionic gonadotrophin

membranoproliferative glomerulonephritis, focal segmental glomerulosclerosis
- Rarely, other types of glomerulonephritis.

Causes of secondary nephrotic syndrome are diabetic nephropathy, drugs (captopril, gold, penicillamine, non-steroidal anti-inflammatory drugs (NSAIDs)), amyloidosis, sickle-cell disease, malaria and vasculitis (systemic lupus erythematosus (SLE)).

Diagnostic approach
After initial assessment using urine dipstick, specialist investigations are performed to exclude systemic diseases, drugs and toxins as the cause of proteinuria. These are summarized in Figure 6.5.

HYPERURICAEMIA

Hyperuricaemia is an excess of uric acid (end-product of purine degradation) in the blood.

Causes

Causes of hyperuricaemia are:

- Overproduction of uric acid: seen in lymphoma, leukaemia, psoriasis and muscle necrosis
- Reduced excretion of uric acid: seen in gout, chronic renal failure (CRF) and hyperparathyroidism
- Drugs: cytotoxins and thiazide diuretics.

Diagnostic approach

Investigation of hyperuricaemia is summarized in Figure 6.6.

DISORDERS OF SERUM SODIUM AND POTASSIUM

Hyponatraemia

In hyponatraemia, plasma [Na^+] is <130 mmol/L and there is a decreased solute:water ratio in the extracellular fluid.

Causes

The causes of hyponatraemia are:

- Diuretics (mainly thiazides)
- Water overload or retention

- Increased antidiuretic hormone (ADH) secretion
- Increased plasma osmolarity (e.g. caused by mannitol, glucose)
- Increased protein or lipids (pseudohyponatraemia). Here, there is less sodium relative to the increase in protein or lipids, giving the impression of a low sodium.

Diagnostic approach

The diagnostic approach to hyponatraemia is shown in Figure 6.7.

Hypernatraemia

In hypernatraemia the serum sodium is >140 mmol/L and there is an increase in solute to water ratio in body fluids and increased serum osmolality (>300 mOsmol/kg).

Causes

The causes of hypernatraemia are:

- Osmotic diuresis (e.g. uncontrolled diabetes)
- Fluid loss without replacement (sweating, burns, vomiting)
- Diabetes insipidus (suspect if lots of dilute urine is produced)
- Incorrect intravenous fluid replacement (i.e. hypertonic fluids)
- Primary aldosteronism.

Diagnostic approach

The diagnostic approach to hypernatraemia is shown in Figure 6.8.

Hypokalaemia

In hypokalaemia plasma [K^+] is <3.5 mmol/L.

Causes

Hypokalaemia is caused by:

- Renal losses due to diuretics, excess mineralocorticoids (Conn's syndrome), magnesium deficiency, renal tubular defects (e.g. renal tubular acidosis), reduced intake or metabolic alkalosis (e.g. vomiting)
- Extrarenal losses due to diarrhoea, laxative abuse, vomiting (pyloric stenosis), profuse sweating, colonic villous adenoma or biliary drainage

Fig. 6.6 Investigation of hyperuricaemia. *Both a xanthine oxidase inhibitor and a uricosuric agent are needed in tophaceous gout. Xanthine oxidase is an enzyme in the metabolic pathway that produces urate from purines. GFR, glomerular filtration rate (from Green HL 1996 Clinical medicine, 2nd edn. Mosby Year Book).

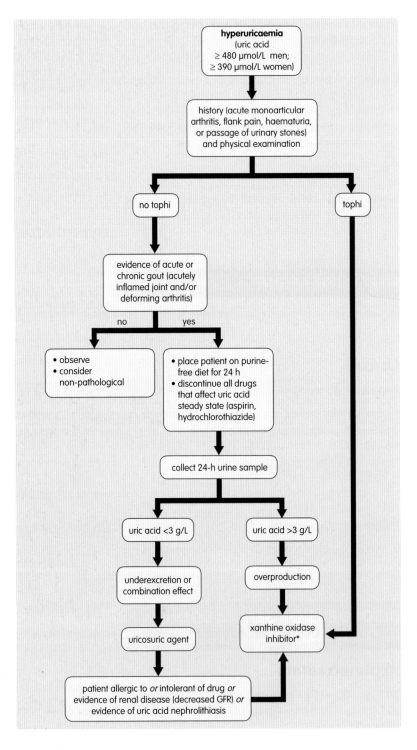

- Transcellular shift due to insulin, metabolic alkalosis, catecholamines and other sympathomimetics, rapid proliferation of cells (e.g. treatment of pernicious anaemia with vitamin B_{12}), or periodic paralysis.

Diagnostic approach

An algorithm for the investigation of hypokalaemia is shown in Figure 6.9.

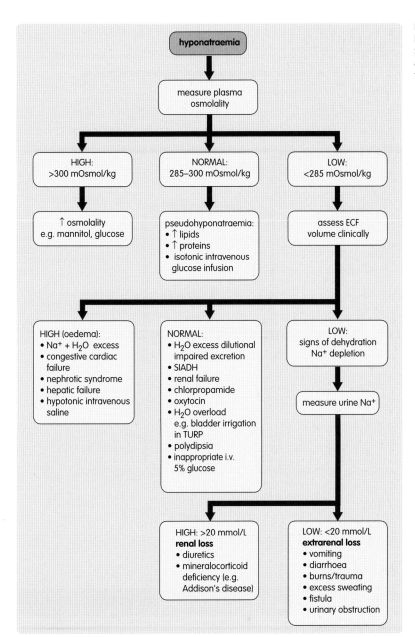

Fig. 6.7 Diagnostic approach to hyponatraemia. ECF, extracellular fluid; SIADH, syndrome of inappropriate antidiuretic hormone secretion; TURP, transurethral resection of the prostate.

Hyperkalaemia

In hyperkalaemia, plasma $[K^+]$ >5.5 mmol/L.

Causes

Hyperkalaemia can result from:

- Reduced renal excretion: due to renal failure, mineralocorticoid deficiency (e.g. Addison's disease), potassium-sparing diuretics or renal tubular defects

- Increased plasma load due to dietary changes or cellular tissue breakdown
- Transcellular shift due to metabolic acidosis, insulin deficiency, exercise or drugs (e.g. digoxin)
- Pseudohyperkalaemia due to efflux from cells (e.g. trauma during venepuncture, prolonged storage, haemolysis), thrombolysis or leucocytosis.

Fig. 6.8 Diagnostic approach to hypernatraemia.

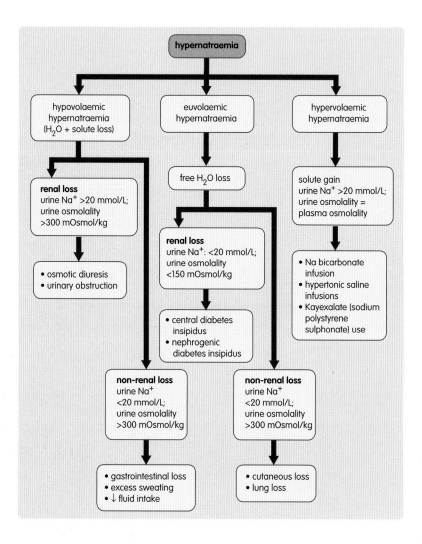

Diagnostic approach

An algorithm for the investigation of hyperkalaemia is shown in Figure 6.10.

The clinical effects of potassium imbalance can be very dangerous. Severe hypokalaemia, (<2.5 mmol/L) requires urgent treatment to prevent hyperpolarization of nerve and muscle cells. This manifests as muscle weakness, hypotonia, cramps and tetany. Cardiac arrhythmias may develop in hypo- *and* hyperkalaemia in which sudden death can result. K+ levels above 6.5 mmol/L require urgent treatment.

RENAL FAILURE

Uraemia

'Uraemia' is the term given to the clinical symptoms which arise when nitrogenous metabolic waste products accumulate in the blood (i.e. urea and creatinine), as a result of decreased filtration of these products by the kidneys. Uraemia may affect any of the body's systems.

- ARF: develops rapidly over hours or a few days and may be reversible.
- CRF: gradual onset over a period of months to years associated with irreversible structural damage within the kidney.

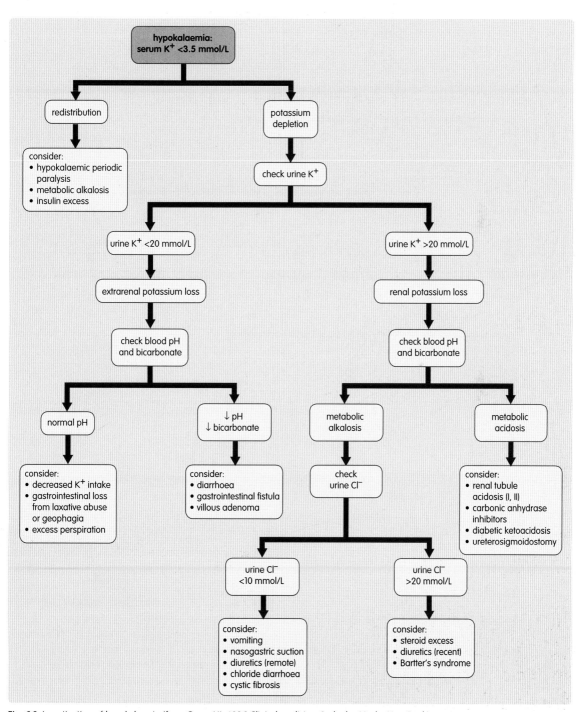

Fig. 6.9 Investigation of hypokalaemia (from Green HL 1996 Clinical medicine, 2nd edn. Mosby Year Book).

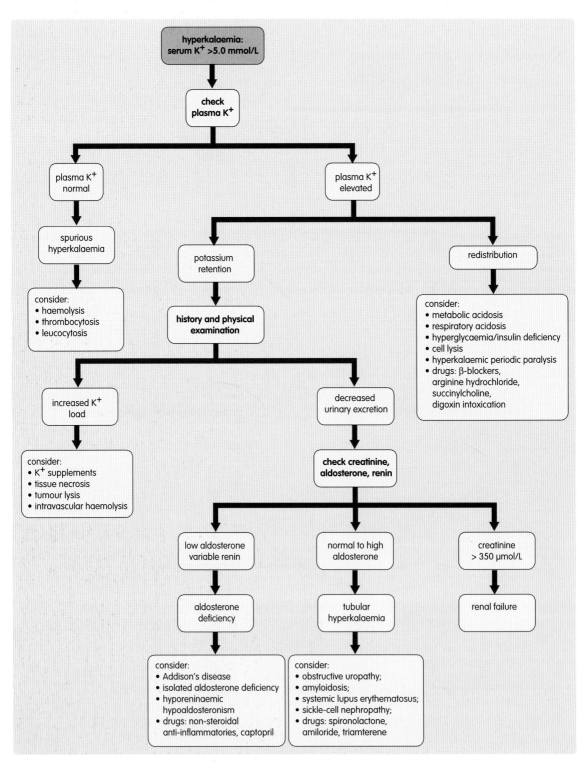

Fig. 6.10 Investigation of hyperkalaemia (from Green HL 1996 Clinical medicine, 2nd edn. Mosby Year Book).

Acute renal failure

Causes of ARF can be classified as prerenal, renal and postrenal.

Prerenal causes of ARF are:

- Hypovolaemia (e.g. shock, burns, dehydration, sepsis, haemorrhage), resulting in decreased effective circulating volume
- Reduced effective circulating volume (e.g. in congestive cardiac failure, liver disease)
- Drugs altering renal haemodynamics (e.g. NSAIDs, angiotensin-converting enzyme inhibitors (ACE), antihypertensives, ciclosporin)
- Renal artery stenosis or emboli.

Renal causes of ARF are:

- Acute tubular necrosis: any untreated prerenal cause, drug toxicity (e.g. gentamicin, aciclovir, methotrexate) and toxins (e.g. myoglobinuria and lipopolysaccharide in Gram-negative sepsis)
- Acute glomerulonephritis
- Acute interstitial nephritis (due to drugs, infections, hypercalcaemia, multiple myeloma)
- Vasculitis
- Hypertension
- Emboli (such as thrombi, cholesterol)
- Acute cortical necrosis (severe shock left untreated).

Postrenal or obstructive causes of ARF are:

- Bladder outflow obstruction (benign prostatic hypertrophy or urethral strictures)
- Retroperitoneal fibrosis
- Tumour (prostate, bladder, or extrinsic compression by gynaecological malignancy)
- Stone (would need to be bilateral to cause ARF).

Note: Obstruction must occur in both kidneys or in a single functioning kidney for renal failure to occur.

Diagnostic approach

First it is important to ask:

- *Is the renal failure acute or chronic?* A history of chronic ill health or signs of chronic renal failure such as anaemia may indicate chronicity, as does small kidneys on ultrasound.
- *Is there urinary tract obstruction?* Obstruction should always be considered as a cause because it is reversible and prompt treatment may prevent permanent renal damage.

- *Is there a rare cause of ARF?* For example, myeloma, systemic vasculitis, haemolytic uraemic syndrome because prompt treatment can be lifesaving.

Basic investigation of renal failure includes urine tests (dipstick, microscopy, culture, cytology), blood tests and renal imaging (KUB (X-ray of the kidney, ureter and bladder), a chest X-ray and an ultrasound of the renal tract). In ARF, the following biochemical changes occur:

- Increased plasma urea and creatinine concentrations
- Increased plasma urate
- Increased plasma concentrations of potassium
- Metabolic acidosis and an increased anion gap
- Increased plasma phosphate and decreased plasma calcium (less marked than in CRF)
- Decreased plasma sodium can occur
- Changes in urine biochemistry: these depend on whether prerenal or renal failure exists (Fig. 6.11).

In addition, some serological tests can help clarify the diagnosis:

- Antinuclear antibodies (ANA): SLE-associated nephritis.
- Cryoglobulin titre: cryoglobulinaemia.
- Complement levels: SLE-associated nephritis, membranoproliferative and acute glomerulonephritis.

Fig. 6.11 Urine biochemistry results

Test	Prerenal failure	Renal failure (acute tubular necrosis)
urine osmolality (mOsm/kg H_2O)	>500	<350
urine sodium (mmol/L)	<20	>40
urine/serum creatinine	>40	<20
urine/serum osmolality	>1.5	<1.2
fractional excreted sodium	<1	>1
renal failure index	↑ urea	↑ urea
	>creatinine	↑ creatinine

Fig. 6.12 Clues to help in diagnosis of acute renal failure and its possible causes

	Prerenal failure	Renal failure	Postrenal failure
History	thirst; weight loss; potential for volume loss (e.g. surgery, diuretics); ineffective circulating volume	previous abnormal urinalysis; exposure to toxic agents; hypertension; new medications	frequency; hesitancy; nocturia; history of nephrolithiasis or neoplasms; renal colic especially if only one kidney
Physical examination	signs of dehydration: hypotension; hypovolaemia; ↓ BP = postural drop; ↑ pulse; ↓ jugular venous pulse	hypertension; physical signs (e.g. skin lesions of vasculitis)	distended bladder; enlarged prostate
Urinalysis	↑ urine osmolality and high specific gravity; ↓urine Na^+ and fractional excreted Na^+; ↑ urine:serum creatinine	proteinuria; haematuria; pyuria; renal tubular epithelial cells in urinary sediment; casts and their nature	crystalluria (suggests renal calculus)

- Antineutrophil cytoplasmic antibodies (ANCA): vasculitis (Wegener's granulomatosis or polyangiitis).

Figure 6.12 gives clues to help in the diagnosis of ARF and its possible causes.

Management

It is important to ensure the patient is adequately resuscitated with appropriate fluid replacement and that adequate nutrition is maintained. It may also be necessary to treat any life-threatening complications urgently (e.g. hyperkalaemia, pulmonary oedema, bleeding) and then deal with the precipitating cause.

Chronic kidney disease

CKD is defined by the presence of structural and or functional alterations within the kidney. It may (but does not always) lead to irreversible loss of renal function which is termed chronic renal failure (CRF). It can result from renal disease or be secondary to other systemic diseases.

CKD is classified into stages according to the level of glomerular filtration rate (GFR). Usually this is estimated (eGFR), using serum creatinine levels and correcting for age, sex and race of the patient. Figure 6.13 shows the staging and classification of CKD.

Causes

Causes of CKD are:

- **Renal**: glomerulonephritis, chronic pyelonephritis, bladder or urethral obstruction, polycystic kidneys, interstitial nephritis, amyloid, myeloma, renal vascular disease, Alport's syndrome.
- **Extrarenal**: diabetes mellitus, hypertension (especially if accelerated-malignant), heart failure, SLE, gout, hypercalcaemia, renovascular disease (atheroma), vasculitis.
- **Drugs**: gold, penicillamine, ciclosporin, analgesics.

Diagnostic approach

Renal function (eGFR) should be measured annually in all patients in the following risk groups:

Fig. 6.13 Classification of chronic kidney disease according to estimated glomerular filtration rate (eGFR)

Stage	eGFR	Description
1	>90	kidney damage with normal or increased eGFR
2	60–89	kidney damage with mild eGFR fall
3	30–59	moderate fall in eGFR
4	15–29	severe fall in eGFR
5	<15 or RRT	established renal failure

Note: To diagnose stages 1–2 there must also be (non-urological) haematuria or proteinuria or a known renal structural abnormality. RRT, renal replacement therapy

- Vascular disease and heart failure
- Patients on ACE inhibitors
- Hypertension
- Diabetes
- Recurrent UTIs
- Bladder outflow obstruction
- Patients maintained on long-term NSAIDs.

The diagnostic approach to CKD can involve:

- **Urine**: urinalysis (haematuria, glycosuria, proteinuria), microscopy (white cells, eosinophilia, granular casts, red cell casts, red cells), biochemistry (protein or albumin to creatinine ration, urinary electrolytes, osmolality, protein electrophoresis).
- **Blood**: urea and creatinine and eGFR, electrolytes, glucose, calcium (decreased), phosphate (increased), urate (increased), protein, osmolality, full blood count, erythrocyte sedimentation rate (ESR), protein electrophoresis, autoantibody screen, complement components, test for sickle cell disease.
- **Radiology**: ultrasound or CT (to assess kidney size), plain radiography of the abdomen and chest X-ray. Hand radiographs can show evidence of osteodystrophy in advanced cases.
- **Renal biopsy**: consider if kidneys are of normal size and the cause of CKD is not clear from other investigations.

Figure 6.14 shows an algorithm for the investigation of CKD.

The estimated eGFR is calculated using the MDRD (modification of diet in renal disease) from the serum creatinine level, age and sex and race of the patient.

RENAL CALCULI

Overview

Kidney stone disease arises from the formation and movement of stones within the urinary tract. It is more common in males. Different types of stones can form:

- Calcium-containing stones are the most common. They are made of calcium oxalate (spiky), hydroxyapatite, phosphate (smooth and large)
- Uric acid stones (smooth, brown and soft)
- Struvite or infection stones
- Cysteine stones (yellow and crystalline).

There is no relation between the size of the stones and the severity of the symptoms.

Causes

Causes of kidney stones are:
- Hypercalciuria (of which hypercalcaemia is the sole cause)
- Hyperuricosuria (of which hyperuricaemia is the main cause)
- Hyperoxaluria
- Cystinuria
- Infection
- Renal tubular acidosis
- Renal disease (e.g. polycystic kidneys)
- Dehydration: a concentrated urine is produced, which increases the risk of stone formation.

Diagnostic approach

History
Ask about the following:

- Diet: high dietary calcium intake (e.g. milk, cheese), high salt intake (calcium is excreted in

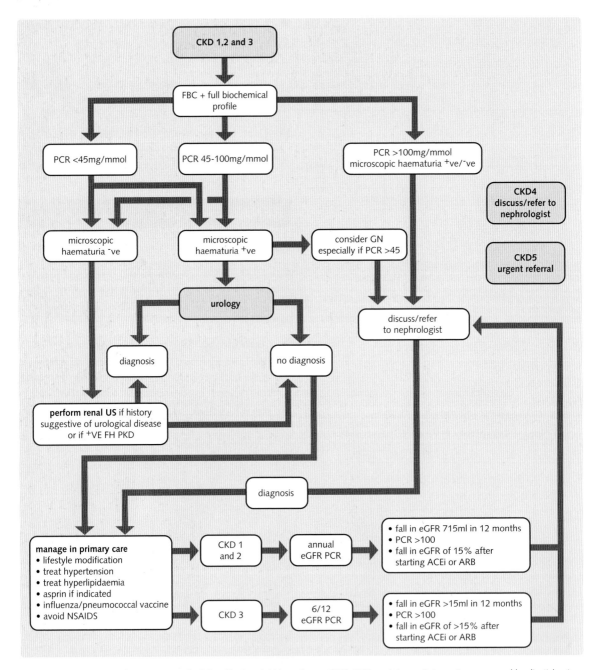

Fig. 6.14 Investigation and management of adults with chronic kidney disease CKD). PCR, protein:creatinine ratio – measured by dipstick urine. Full biochemical profile includes urea and electrolytes, HCO_3^-, albumin, calcium phosphate and alkaline phosphate. FBC, full blood count; GN, glomerulonephritis; US, ultrasound; PKD, polycystic kidney disease; ACEi, angiotensin-converting enzyme inhibitors.

parallel with sodium in the kidney), high dietary oxalate intake (e.g. spinach, rhubarb, tea)
- Fluid intake and urine volume
- Chronic diarrhoea: Crohn's disease or dehydration
- Personal or family history of gout

- Family history of renal calculi
- Number of previous UTIs.
- Medications: check for antacid therapy (contains large amounts of absorbable calcium) and long-term antibiotic therapy
- Past urological history.

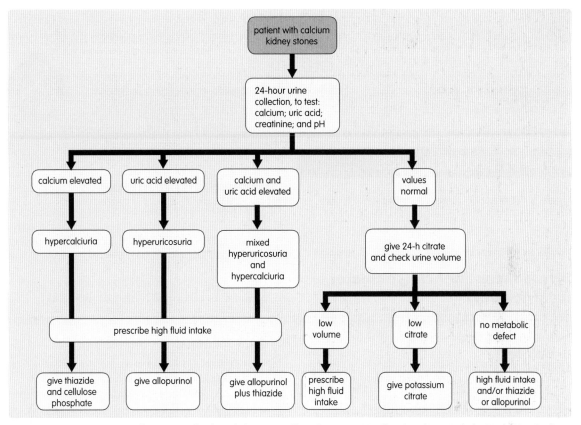

Fig. 6.15 Urinary investigations of a patient with calcium kidney stones (from Green HL 1996 Clinical medicine, 2nd edn. Mosby Year Book).

Symptoms

In acute presentation, pain is usually colicky and localised to one quadrant of the abdomen, radiating from loin to groin. The patient appears sweaty, pale and restless, with nausea and vomiting.

Examination and investigation

Examinations and investigations for renal calculi should include:

- Looking for clinical evidence of gout
- Excluding hypercalcaemia and investigating cause if found (e.g. primary hyperparathyroidism)
- Urinalysis: identify and quantify the amount of calcium, oxalate, urate or cysteine in the urine. Is there any haematuria?
- Stone analysis: ask patient to retain voided stones for biochemical testing or X-ray crystallography
- Imaging: computed tomography (CT) (or magnetic resonance imaging (MRI)) is now the preferred first line investigations for suspected renal calculi. Plain radiographs showing the kidneys, ureters and bladder (KUB), and abdominal ultrasound are also used (may show dilatation of obstructed kidney or acoustic shadow from a stone). Intravenous urography (IVU) may be helpful but cannot be used when renal function is impaired.

Figure 6.15 shows an algorithm for urinary investigations of a patient with calcium kidney stones.

Treatment

Acute episodes are treated with analgesia and increased fluid intake. Urine should be 'sieved' to collect any stones passed for analysis (most pass spontaneously). If obstruction or infection develops, the stones must be removed urgently. In the long term, the mainstay of treatment is a high fluid intake; thiazides can be used in hypercalcuria as they decrease urinary calcium excretion. Allopurinol is used for hyperuricaemia, and penicillamine for cystinuria.

Kidney stones cause loin pain.
Ureteric stones cause renal colic.
Bladder stones cause 'strangulation', i.e. the desire to pass the stone, but being unable to do so by voiding.

URINARY INCONTINENCE

Urinary incontinence is the involuntary loss of urine. It affects more women than men and is a socially distressing condition. There are several different types.

Stress incontinence (sphincter insufficiency)

This is involuntary loss of urine associated with an increase in intra-abdominal pressure (e.g. cough). It is caused by:

- Pelvic floor laxity (usually seen in multiparous women).
- Bladder neck sphincter impairment (more common in middle-aged, obese, multiparous women).
- Surgery affecting the urethra or prostate causing damage or weakness to the external sphincter.

Urge incontinence (detrusor instability)

This is involuntary loss of urine, with the urge to void. There is an urgent 'need to go'. It is due to sensory or motor dysfunction of the bladder. Causes include:

- Inflammation or infection of the lower urinary tract
- Bladder hyper-reflexia
- Stroke
- Parkinson's disease
- Alzheimer's disease
- Brain tumour
- Old age
- Herniated spinal disc
- Detrusor overactivity caused by a foreign body, stone or urethritis
- Benign prostatic hypertrophy and obstruction (can cause bladder hypersensitivity)

- Loop diuretics
- Cough or sneeze.

The detrusor muscle is the bladder muscle and contracts to cause voiding. This is an automatic reflex, triggered by filling of the bladder to a critical pressure.

Overflow incontinence

This is involuntary leakage of urine when the bladder is full. It is usually due to chronic urine retention secondary to obstruction or an atonic bladder. The causes are:

- Outlet obstruction: faecal impaction, benign prostatic hypertrophy (enlarged prostate)
- Underactive detrusor muscle
- Bladder neck stricture
- Urethral stricture
- α-adrenergic agonists
- Intra- or postoperative overdistension
- Use of anticholinergics, calcium channel blockers, sedatives
- Bladder denervation following surgery.

Total incontinence

This is continuous loss of urine with no voluntary control. The causes are:

- Congenital
- Secondary to paraplegia, multiple sclerosis, spina bifida
- Trauma to the external sphincter, bladder neck and perineal muscles
- Fistula secondary to radiation, surgery, tumour, invasive neoplasms, obstetric injury.

Reflex incontinence

This is involuntary intermittent loss of urine.

Functional incontinence

This is incontinence due to severe cognitive impairment or mobility limitations, preventing use of the toilet. For example, there might be difficulty in reaching the toilet or difficulty in undressing, and the patient is 'caught short'. Bladder function is normal.

Mixed incontinence

In mixed incontinence there is more than one type of problem resulting in incontinence. This is usually seen in older patients.

Nocturnal enuresis – bedwetting

Nocturnal enuresis is a childhood disorder. It can be primary (since birth) or secondary (acquired). Both can be due to:

- Uninhibited bladder activity
- Urinary infection
- Neurological disease
- Obstruction.

After urinary tract infection has been excluded, no further investigation should be performed if the child is under 5 years – unless there are any urinary symptoms. Treatment should focus on behaviour therapy, with drug treatment used only as a last resort – sublingual desmopressin is one example.

Diagnostic approach

Figure 6.16 shows an algorithm for the investigation of urinary incontinence.

URINARY TRACT INFECTION

Overview

Urinary tract infection (UTI) (i.e. $>10^5$ organisms/mL) occurs with or without leucocytes. It is more common in adult females because bacteria can readily access the urinary tract through the short female urethra. UTI results from migration of bacteria through the urethra into the bladder, ureter and kidney. UTIs are also seen in male infants with congenital obstruction and in elderly men with acquired prostatic obstruction. Different sites of the urinary tract can be affected as follows:

- Upper urinary tract: kidney, resulting in pyelonephritis
- Lower urinary tract: bladder, resulting in cystitis; prostate, resulting in prostatitis; urethra, resulting in urethritis.

Risk factors for UTI are:

- Diabetes mellitus
- Pregnancy

- Impaired voiding (due to obstruction)
- Genitourinary malformations
- Sexual intercourse
- Stones
- Neurogenic bladder
- Intact male foreskin.

The main organisms involved are:

- *Escherichia coli* (>70% of cases)
- *Staphylococcus saprophyticus*
- *Proteus* species
- *Klebsiella* species
- *Enterobacter* species
- *Pseudomonas* species
- *Enterococcus* species

A urinary tract infection in children must always be investigated to exclude vesicoureteric reflux, which can lead to kidney scarring and hypertension.

Diagnostic approach

Algorithms for the investigation of UTI are given in Figures 6.17 and 6.18.

OTHER PRESENTATIONS OF DISEASES OF THE RENAL TRACT

Urethral discharge

A urethral discharge is secretion passed through the urethra at times other than voiding. The female equivalent is vaginal discharge. The secretion may be clear, purulent, bloody, itchy or foul smelling.

Causes

Causes of urethral discharge are:

- Non-infectious: irritation (mechanical or chemical), urethral stricture, non-bacterial prostatitis, phimosis, urethral diverticulum, urethral carbuncle. Occasionally, it can be caused by Reiter's syndrome.
- Infectious (i.e. sexually transmitted infections): gonococcal urethritis (characteristically 'canary

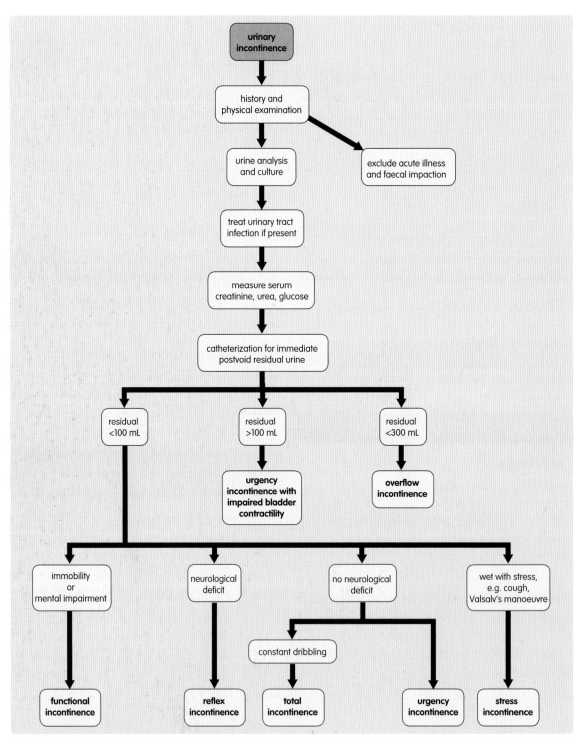

Fig. 6.16 Investigation of urinary incontinence. UTI, urinary tract infection (from Green HL 1996 Clinical medicine, 2nd edn. Mosby Year Book).

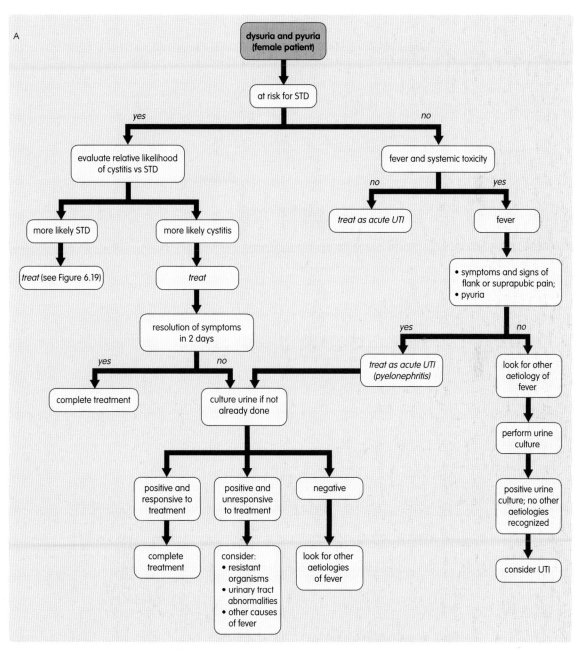

Fig. 6.17 A Investigation of urinary tract infection. Dysuria and pyuria in a female patient. STD, sexually transmitted disease; UTI, urinary tract infection (from Green HL 1996 Clinical medicine, 2nd edn. Mosby Year Book).

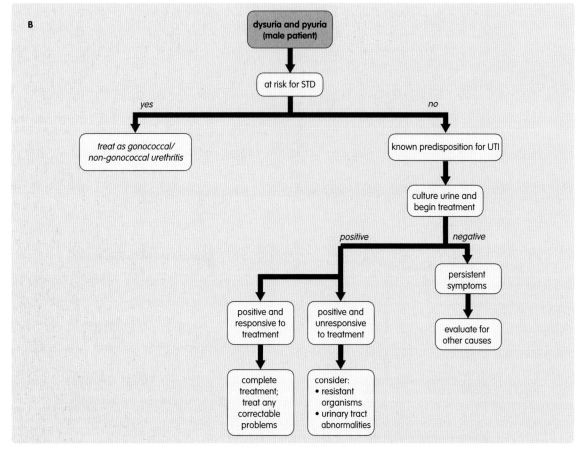

Fig. 6.17 B Dysuria and pyuria in a male patient. STD, sexually transmitted disease; UTI, urinary tract infection (from Green HL 1996 Clinical medicine, 2nd edn. Mosby Year Book).

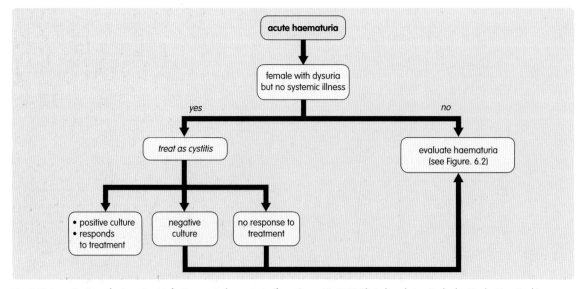

Fig. 6.18 Investigation of urinary tract infection: acute haematuria (from Green HL 1996 Clinical medicine, 2nd edn. Mosby Year Book).

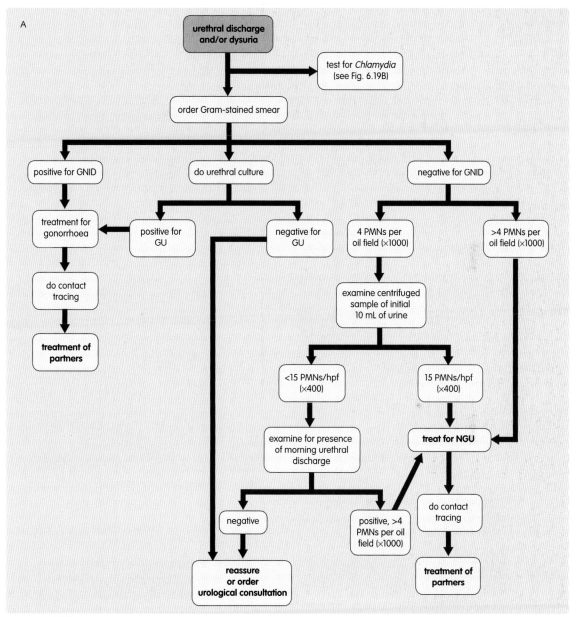

Fig. 6.19 A Diagnosing urethral discharge. GNID, Gram-negative intracellular diplococci; GU, gonococcal urethritis; hpf, high-power field; NGU, non-gonococcal urethritis; PMNs, polymorphonuclear leucocytes (from Green HL 1996 Clinical medicine, 2nd edn. Mosby Year Book).

yellow' discharge) or, more commonly, non-gonococcal urethritis (i.e. *Chlamydia trachomatis, Trichomonas vaginalis,* herpes simplex virus).

Diagnostic approach

An algorithm for diagnosing urethral discharge is given in Figure 6.19.

Dysfunctional voiding

In dysfunctional voiding there are abnormal characteristics of voiding. It is important to find out how the symptoms differ from normal for the patient. They can be:

- Irritative: producing frequency, nocturia, urgency and dysuria

Fig. 6.19 B Investigation for *Chlamydia trachomatis*.

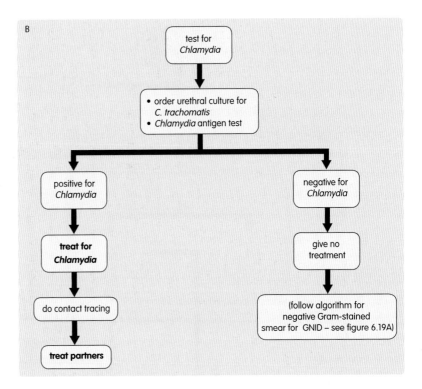

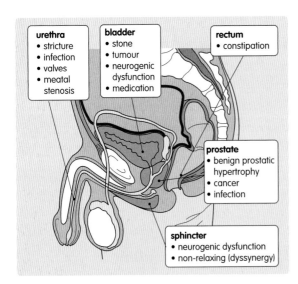

Fig. 6.20 Causes of obstructive bladder symptoms.

- Obstructive: producing hesitancy, diminished force, dribbling and increased residual urine.

Causes

Irritative bladder symptoms can be caused by:

- Local abnormality with decreased bladder capacity: this can be the result of infection, inflammation or fibrosis. Causes include acute pyogenic infections, chronic infections (i.e. tuberculosis), chlamydia, chronic fungi, foreign body, stones, trauma, radiation, cyclophosphamide, interstitial cystitis and chronic obstruction.
- Neurological abnormality: this can be the result of stroke, cerebral atrophy or multiple sclerosis, all of which damage the cortex or upper spinal cord.

Obstructive bladder symptoms are more common in men because they have a longer urethra, which is easily compressed or narrowed. Causes are summarized in Figure 6.20.

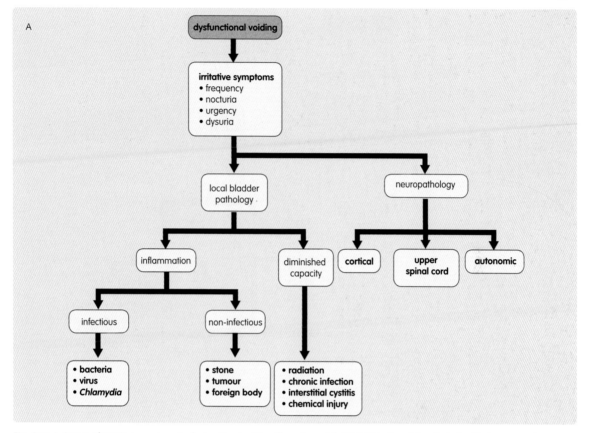

A

Fig. **6.21** A Causes of irritative symptoms in dysfunctional voiding (from Green HL 1996 Clinical medicine, 2nd edn. Mosby Year Book).

Diagnostic approach

A comparison of the aetiology of irritative and obstructive bladder symptoms in dysfunctional voiding is shown in Figure 6.21.

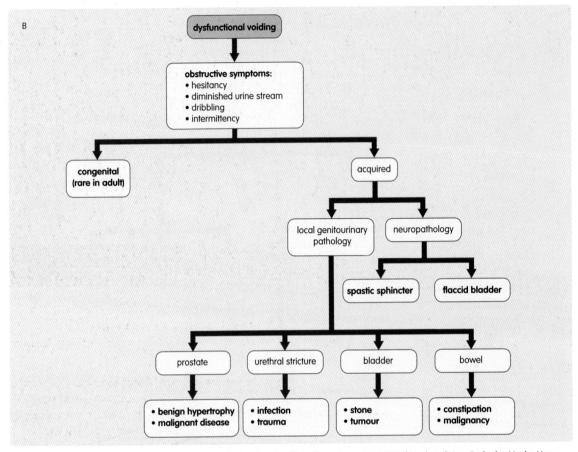

Fig. 6.21 B Causes of obstructive bladder symptoms in dysfunctional voiding (from Green HL 1996 Clinical medicine, 2nd edn. Mosby Year Book).

History and examination

Objectives

By the end of this chapter you should be able to:

- Describe which symptoms are particularly relevant to the urinary system
- Briefly describe the skills required to conduct an effective consultation
- List what you might see around a patient to help you assess the patient's condition
- Describe the clinical signs associated with renal disease
- Explain how to measure the blood pressure
- List the possible findings on auscultation of the heart in renal disease
- Describe how to examine the kidneys
- List the possible causes for unilateral and bilateral kidney enlargement
- Explain how you can test for ascites, and what the renal-related causes are
- Outline the possible findings on digital rectal examination.

TAKING A HISTORY

Overview

A full history is the first and most important step in making the correct diagnosis. Before taking a history, always introduce yourself – shake hands and tell the patient your name and status (i.e. medical student). Explain what you are going to do and make sure that the patient understands. Before you start, check that the patient is comfortable and relaxed.

Stand back and look around the bedside for clues such as inhalers, oxygen mask, dialysis equipment, blood glucose (BM) sticks, walking sticks and frames (indicates restricted mobility), sputum pot, cards from the family (shows support), and reading material. Also, observe the patient – look for any agitation, difficulties in breathing, speech problems, tremors or deafness.

Structure of the history

The following is a basic guide to structuring the history. Start by taking the patient's name, date of birth and occupation.

Presenting complaint

Allow the patient to explain in his or her own words what the problem is and record the symptoms that the patient describes.

History of the presenting complaint

Features of the presenting complaint to ask about include:

- What is the nature of the complaint? Find out about the symptom, e.g. for pain ask about site, radiation, severity, timing, character (stabbing, burning, pricking), aggravating or relieving factors, and associated symptoms.
- What is the onset and time-course of the complaint? Did the symptom occur gradually or suddenly? When did it begin? Is there a pattern and, if so, what? Find out whether the symptom is intermittent or constant, how frequently it occurs, how long it lasts for and its intensity.
- Are there any precipitating or relieving factors? Does anything bring it on, make it worse or better (e.g. position, food, pain killers)? In renal colic, the patient will not be comfortable in any position and is constantly moving and writhing.
- Are there other relevant or associated symptoms, e.g. if the presenting complaint is loin pain, ask about urinary frequency, blood in urine, nausea or vomiting, constipation or diarrhoea.
- Has the patient had any previous treatment or investigations for this complaint? Has the patient had a similar problem before and what was done about it?

Symptoms relevant to the urinary system are:

- Haematuria (cancer of the renal tract, urinary tract infection, glomerulonephritis)

- Increased frequency (urinary tract infection)
- Poor stream (bladder outflow obstruction – prostatic hypertrophy)
- Nocturia (chronic renal failure or bladder outflow obstruction).

Past medical history

Find out about any illnesses, operations, investigations and treatments, with dates. Elicit the details of past or current medical conditions, such as tuberculosis, asthma, heart conditions, previous strokes, jaundice and epilepsy. Ask about medical conditions associated with renal disease (e.g. diabetes mellitus, hypertension, chronic inflammatory disease, cancer, urinary tract infections, rheumatic fever, tonsillitis and previous renal disease). Make a note of any recent infections – in particular, streptococcal throat infections, as this can trigger post-infective glomerulonephritis.

Obstetric and gynaecological history

Ask about any prolonged labour (resulting in lax pelvic floor muscles), caesarean sections or pelvic inflammatory disease.

Drug history

Determine if the patient:

- Is taking any medications – ask about prescribed and over-the-counter drugs
- Has any known allergies (e.g. penicillin)
- Has been exposed to any toxins (e.g. industrial toxins, lead and hydrocarbons).

Family history

Note any known medical conditions in first-degree relatives – in particular, renal disease, hypertension and diabetes. Draw a concise diagram of the family tree.

Social history

It is also important to find out the patient's social circumstances. Enquire about the patient's:

- Marital status: children and spouse's health.
- Occupation: current job or past job, effect of illness on job, financial problems.
- Accommodation: where does the patient live and who with? Are there any relatives or friends visiting? Can the patient cope at home (i.e. cooking, washing, home surroundings)?
- Diet and exercise.
- Travel: has the patient been abroad recently?
- Alcohol: how many units does the patient drink? (The best way to assess this is to go

through the weekly consumption with the patient.)
- Smoking: how much? When did the patient start? If they are an ex-smoker, establish how many years they smoked, how many a day and for how long they have given up.
- Drugs: 'recreational' drugs. How much? How often? For how long?
- Sexual practices.

Systems review

This is a brief overview of all the body systems (Fig. 7.1).

Summary

Always end with a short summary including:

- The name, age and occupation of the patient
- The presenting complaint and its duration
- Any relevant associated symptoms or medical history.

> Always ask about occupation, as in patients exposed to carcinogens, renal disease may develop or existing renal disease may worsen.

Communication skills

Effective doctor–patient communication is the basis of accurate history taking, correct diagnosis and successful management. As well as improving the patient's experience of medical care, it offers reassurance and can reduce anxiety. Poor communication can lead to poor compliance, dissatisfaction and mistrust. Ideas and understanding about illness and its implications can vary according to the patient's background and beliefs, so it is important to establish these and develop a care plan that accommodates the patient's needs. Often, a third party will be involved in the patient's care, for example:

- Elderly patients: their carers
- Children: their parents
- Patients from a different ethnic background: an interpreter (possibly another family member)
- Patients who are deaf or blind: an interpreter.

In these cases, clear questioning and explanations are critical to ensure both the patient and the

Fig. 7.1 Summary of systems review

General/body system	Examination
general questions	weight loss (carcinoma) appetite night sweats fevers (infections) lumps (carcinoma) fatigue (carcinoma)
genitourinary	**incontinence** **dysuria** **haematuria** **nocturia** **frequency** **polyuria** **hesitancy** **dribbling** menstrual history (cycle and duration, regularity, first day of last menstrual period, number of pregnancies, menarche and menopause)
cardiorespiratory	chest pain (heart disease) dyspnoea palpitations (heart disease) paroxysmal nocturnal dyspnoea ankle oedema (Na^+ and water retention) cough and sputum haemoptysis wheeze (asthma)
gastrointestinal	abdominal pain nausea and vomiting (uraemia) bowel frequency tenesmus or urgency malaena (carcinoma) haematemesis flatulence dysphagia
neurological	**fits, blackouts** **headaches** **sphincter disturbances** **dizziness**
musculoskeletal and skin	pain swelling of joints gout **rashes/skin conditions**

Note: Bold indicates those examinations especially relevant to the renal and urinary systems

accompanying third party understand what is happening.

When taking a history or examination, always consider the following points:

- Structure the consultation in a logical manner, modifying it to accommodate the patient's needs.

- Appear confident and at ease to reassure the patient. Over 60% of communication is non-verbal, so factors such as posture and eye contact have a significant role in conveying your feelings to the patient.
- Position yourself so you sit facing the patient at the same level. This implies equality – never treat the patient as inferior to you.
- Start with open questions, and then ask closed questions to obtain specific answers. Find out the patient's understanding of the nature of the problem, and his or her perception of what treatment will involve.
- Listen actively and encourage the patient to talk. Actions such as nodding, smiling or echoing the patient's last sentence can help him or her to relax and shows that you are listening. This in turn can prompt the patient to expand on points.
- Allow pauses to encourage the patient to talk further, and to digest what is being said.
- Respond to any concerns that the patient might have and check that the patient understands what is going to happen next.
- Avoid jargon or technical language.
- At the end of the consultation, repeat what the patient has told you to check that you have obtained the correct information, and to clarify any points.

Patient care also involves liaising between many different hospital and community healthcare workers, which again depends on clear communication between these groups.

- Use open questions to establish the patient's beliefs.
- Use closed questions to obtain and classify facts to narrow down the patient's diagnosis.

HISTORY TAKING SUMMARY

In practise, when taking a history, you may not get much time and it will be necessary to focus on the key points outlined in this section.

Presenting complaint:

- Record main symptoms.

History of presenting complaint

- Expand on symptoms
- Similar previous problems/treatments?

Past medical history

- Any conditions associated with renal disease?
- All illnesses
- All operations
- All investigations
- All treatments.

Drug history

- Current medication
- Any allergies – drugs or otherwise.

Family history

First-degree relatives – conditions, particularly renal disease.

Social history

- Marital status
- Occupation
- Accommodation
- Recent travel
- Alcohol
- Smoking.

GENERAL INSPECTION

Overview

Whenever you examine a patient it is important to remember the following points:

- Always introduce yourself to the patient.
- Observe the patient carefully before you begin the examination to gain an overall impression of the patient's condition.
- Look around the patient for any extra clues – dialysis equipment, sputum pot or oxygen mask.
- Position the patient appropriately for the examination – at 45 degrees for cardiovascular or respiratory system examination or lying flat for abdominal examination.
- Expose the appropriate part of body only and ensure the patient is comfortable.
- Observe the patient from the end of the bed before you start the examination.
- Notice if the patient is conscious or looks well, is in pain, appears anxious or depressed, smells of urine or has any obvious skeletal abnormalities.
- Look at the patient's stature (Fig. 7.2), any obvious skin pigmentation (Fig. 7.3) and fat distribution.
- The fluid status of the patient should be noted. Useful physical signs include:

Fig. 7.2 Tests for signs related to stature and weight in renal disease		
Test	**Sign**	**Diagnostic inference**
observe patient's stature	short stature	seen in patients who had CRF in childhood: growth is impaired due to an abnormal response to growth hormone and puberty is delayed
calculate BMI: BMI = weight/height^2 and compare with ideal BMI	underweight : BMI <19 kg/m^2 or overweight : BMI >30 kg/m^2 an increase in weight can be due to oedema	• oedema of nephrotic syndrome can be confused with obesity • a low BMI is seen in CRF due to anorexia and malnutrition
check for oedema by pressing tissues with thumb and looking for a pit left in the tissues	• periorbital oedema (swelling of the eyelid) • general puffiness of the face • oedema of the legs • sacral oedema • ascites	renal causes of oedema: • acute glomerulonephritis • nephrotic syndrome • renal failure

Note: BMI, body mass index; CRF, chronic renal failure

Fig. 7.3 Tests for signs related to skin colour in renal disease

Test	Sign	Diagnostic inference
observe the patient's skin and eyes, looking for any changes, such as pallor	conjunctivae are pale	in CRF, there is a decrease in erythropoietin causing an anaemia with normal iron concentration; other causes of anaemia are iron, vitamin B_{12} and folate deficiency
observe the patient's skin and eyes, looking for any changes, such as bruising	areas of skin that are blue/black in colour	in CRF, the bleeding time is increased, leading to bleeding in tissues
observe the patient's skin and eyes, looking for any changes, such as pigmentation	areas of darkened skin on either the face or limbs; pale yellow tinge to skin	increased production of melanin-stimulating hormone causes melanin deposition in the skin; also, urochrome deposition in the skin
observe the patient's skin and eyes, looking for any changes, such as polycythaemia	red and rugged appearance of the face	sign of polycythaemia occasionally seen in: • polycystic kidneys • post-transplant • carcinoma of the kidney

Note: CRF, chronic renal failure

- elevated jugular venous pressure (JVP)
- pleural effusion
- pulmonary oedema
- peripheral pitting oedema (most prominent at the ankles and sacrum).
- Signs indicating that the patient is on dialysis include the presence of a dialysis machine, fistula or continuous ambulatory peritoneal dialysis catheter. These indicate that the patient is in acute or end-stage renal failure, treated by dialysis.

Face and neck signs related to renal disease are listed in Figure 7.4.

HANDS AND LIMBS

Abnormalities of the nails that indicate underlying renal disease are summarized in Figure 7.5. To examine the hands, spread out the fingers on a flat, white surface. This will highlight any shortening of the distal phalanges; a difference of length between the fingers is often seen in severe renal osteo-dystrophy secondary to chronic renal failure. This is due to chronic high circulating levels of parathyroid hormone. The patient should then hold the hands straight out to the front. Watch for any movement – this can be detected more easily by putting a piece of paper on top of the hands. If a coarse 'dipping' movement is noted in the outstretched fingers, which is exaggerated by wrist dorsiflexion, the possible diagnosis is severe uraemia, a preterminal sign in patients with renal disease that indicates the need for immediate dialysis.

However, this cannot be distinguished from any of the other metabolic flaps (asterixis) caused by:

- CO_2 retention in respiratory failure
- Chronic liver disease.

Changes in the limbs in renal disease are listed in Figure 7.6.

THORAX

Respiratory system

Few signs in a respiratory examination indicate renal disease. The key change to watch for is the pattern and rate of respiration – patients with a metabolic acidosis associated with chronic renal failure often have a deep, sigh-like respiration, with a rapid breathing rate. This is known as Kussmaul's

Fig. 7.4 Signs in the face and neck related to renal disease

Test	Sign	Diagnostic inference
polycythaemia	red and rugged appearance of the face	sign of polycythaemia occasionally seen in: • polycystic kidneys • post-transplant • carcinoma of the kidney
look for deposits on forehead	white powdery crystals of urate look like dandruff on the forehead	sign of uraemic frost – the crystals form from excess urea in the sweat and are a terminal sign of CRF
look for deposits in the sclera	yellow deposits in the sclera	calcium deposits due to hyperparathyroidism
look for retinal changes	retinal changes typical of diabetes, hypertension and vascular disease	seen in: • diabetes mellitus • hypertension • vascular disease
check hearing	deafness	Alport syndrome
look at mucous membranes of mouth	ulceration of the mouth and lips	severely ill patients (impaired immune system)
look at mucous membranes of mouth	white deposit in the mouth of fungal infection	patients on cytotoxic drugs or steroids; immunosuppression with drugs can result in opportunistic infections such as candidal infection
be aware of patients's breath	halitosis (bad breath), either: • ammonia smell • acetone smell	respectively due to: • renal failure • ketoacidosis

Note: CRF, chronic renal failure

Fig. 7.5 Nail signs in renal disease

Test	Sign	Diagnostic inference
look for markings on nail	transverse ridges (Beau's lines)	indicative of: • past malnutrition • severe illness
	splinter haemorrhages	renal failure due to: • vasculitis (e.g. Wegener's granulomatosis) • bacterial endocarditis
look for discoloration of nails	brown discoloration of nails	CRF
	opaque with discoloration of the nails	nephrotic syndrome and CRF

Note: CRF, chronic renal failure

respiration, and is caused by direct stimulation of the respiratory centre in an attempt to correct the systemic acidosis. A similar respiratory pattern is seen in severe untreated diabetic ketoacidosis.

Cardiovascular system

Blood pressure

Many patients with renal disease will have an elevated blood pressure. When measuring blood

Fig. 7.6 Changes in the limbs in renal disease

Test	Sign	Diagnostic inference
observe appearance and texture of skin	dry flaky skin	CRF
	scratch marks and bruises on limbs and abdomen	uraemic pruritus due to hyperphosphataemia and dry skin
	dirty brown appearance which can make the patient look very healthy or tanned	CRF causing an increase in photosensitive pigment (pseudoporphyrin) as a result of decreased clearance of porphyrins in the urine and increased melanin secondary to increased MSH
look for skin scars or lesions	fistulae are often seen on the forearm	fistulae allow access to blood at a high pressure for haemodialysis
	scars from previous surgically constructed fistulae	vascular access clots and often needs reconstruction
look for deformities of bones and joints; check range of movement, signs of inflammation and for any pain	valgus (knock knees) and varus (bow legs) deformities	renal rickets due to renal osteodystrophy
	painful, inflammed and red	acute gout due to the deposition of urate crystals in joints
look for any involuntary movement	sporadic twitching of limbs (often accompanies a tremor)	indicative of need for immediate renal replacement therapy
	some patients have an uncontrollable need to move their limbs all the time (restless limbs)	CRF or on dialysis
measure blood pressure	postural drop in BP	hypovolaemia
look for oedema: pitting if there is indentation of the skin after 10 s of finger pressure	generalized swelling of limb and pitting; if present at ankle, check at knee and mid-thigh	pitting oedema is characteristic of: • fluid overload due to salt and water retention • nephrotic syndrome • congestive cardiac failure
look for rash	purpuric rash (cutaneous haemorrhage)	vasculitis (e.g. Henoch–Schönlein purpura)
check skin and subcutaneous tissue turgor: assessed by rolling a pinch of soft tissue between finger and thumb	the skin will seem less elastic and tense	skin and subcutaneous turgor is reduced in: • old age • Na$^+$ depletion • malnutrition
test peripheral sensation	a glove and stocking distribution of peripheral sensory loss, indicating peripheral neuropathy	advanced renal failure (rare)

Note: BP, blood pressure; MSH, melanocyte-stimulating hormone; CRF, chronic renal failure

pressure (which needs to be done on several occasions) it is important to measure it on the same limb each time to ensure consistent and comparable results. To ensure measurement is accurate:

• Select the correct cuff size
• Use the cuff on a fully extended arm with the stethoscope applied lightly to the brachial artery
• Always take the blood pressure with the patient sitting and standing. This is because a 5–10 mmHg increase in diastolic pressure is usually seen on standing in a patient with a healthy cardiovascular system (CVS). Postural hypotension (i.e. a drop in diastolic pressure on standing) can be detected only if both measurements are made.

The World Health Organization (WHO) defines hypertension as maintained systolic pressure of 140 mmHg or above and a diastolic pressure of

Fig. 7.7 Superficial findings in the cardiovascular system in renal disease

Test	Sign	Diagnostic inference
look for abnormality of chest wall	increased curvature of spine and rounded shoulders	softening of vertebrae due to renal osteodystrophy in the spine (rugger jersey spine on radiograph)
look for scars: note position on chest and check round to back following the ribs	midline scars old scars are white and pale and recent scars are purple–red in colour	previous heart surgery
jugular venous pressure (an indicator of internal fluid load): the patient should be at 45° and with head turned away from you; note any pulsations in the internal jugular vein	normally jugular venous pulse is not visible, but can be seen by occluding the vein just above the clavicle if a waveform is visible then measure the height from the top of the fluid level vertically down to the angle of Louis	jugular venous pressure is raised in: • right heart failure • fluid overload • chronic bronchitis

Fig. 7.8 Findings on palpation of the cardiovascular system in renal disease

Test	Sign	Diagnostic inference
apex beat is normally felt in the mid-clavicular line at the level of the fifth intercostal space; this is the most lateral point at which the pulsation can be felt – note its position and strength	lateral displacement	left ventricular dilatation causing enlargement of the heart pneumothorax
	impalpable	• obesity • pleural effusion • pericardial effusion
	thrusting and strong	• high blood pressure • left ventricular hypertrophy
peripheral pulses	presence or absence listen with a stethoscope for bruits	atherosclerosis if present may suggest renovascular disease

90 mmHg or above. However, blood pressure levels lower than this are associated with improved survival in epidemiological studies. Most renal diseases are associated with the development of hypertension.

Observation, palpation, percussion and auscultation

Examine the CVS with the patient sitting at 45 degrees and undressed from the waist up. Figure 7.7 summarizes the superficial signs in the CVS in renal disease and Figure 7.8 shows the findings on palpation in the CVS examination. Percussion of the heart borders can be dull beyond the normal boundaries of the mediastinum, which suggests an enlarged heart. Decreased breath sounds at the bases of the lungs indicates pleural effusion, which can occur in:

• Nephrotic syndrome
• Congestive heart failure
• Fluid retention.

The positive findings on auscultation of the CVS are shown in Figure 7.9.

Fig. 7.9 Positive findings on ascultation of the cardiovascular system in renal disease

Test	Sign	Diagnostic inference
heart sounds: listen for audibility, rate and accentuation of the sound in all four areas	muffled and soft	pericardial effusion
	prominent aortic component of the second heart sound	hypertension
	a low-pitched third heart sound heard after the second heart sound	an early sign to left ventricular failure or fluid overload
	gallop rhythm (two normal heart sounds with a third and tachycardia)	• fluid overload • ventricular failure
murmurs: • low pitch (apex) with the bell • high pitch with the diaphragm feel the carotid pulse – time the murmur with the cardiac cycle	• functional murmurs • murmurs due to coexisting valve disease	• aortic and pulmonary regurgitation due to dilatation of the valve ring secondary to fluid overload • mitral regurgitation due to annular calification of the valve; anaemia
pericardial rub: listen carefully over the precordium	a localized or generalized scratchy sound heard in any part of the cardiac cycle heard best if the patient leans forward	this friction rub (two layers of the pericardial layer moving in the presence of an exudate) occurs in: • pericarditis (a terminal feature of CRF) • uraemic pericarditis • systemic lupus erythematosus and vasculitis • intermittent illness in a patient with CRF

Note: CRF, chronic renal failure

ABDOMEN

Overview

The patient should be lying as flat as possible on a firm mattress with arms by the side and head supported with one or two pillows – check that the patient is comfortable. This position ensures that the abdominal muscles are relaxed, making palpation much easier.

Stand on the right-hand side of the bed, ideally with the patient exposed from 'nipples to knees'; to maintain privacy expose the patient from the xiphisternum to the level of the symphysis pubis.

Examination of the genitalia is a vital part of examination of the abdominal system. They should either be covered up once inspection is complete or be examined later. Remember to tell the patient that you will need to examine the genitalia and to perform a rectal examination and (if the patient is female) vaginal examination. A chaperone must be present while conducting genital examinations.

Inspection

Spend the first 20–30 s inspecting the patient from the end of the bed. Look around the patient for any clues – drips, drains and dialysis machines. Figure 7.10 gives the signs usually seen on general inspection of the abdomen in a patient with renal disease.

Palpation

Before palpating, check if the patient is in pain. If the answer is yes, ask where the painful or tender area is and start palpating from the point furthest from the locus of the pain. Tell the patient to breathe normally and relax – you will be able to feel much more through relaxed abdominal muscles. It can help to kneel at the bedside so that you are at the same level as the patient – always demonstrate this in an examination.

Develop a routine for examining all the regions and organs to avoid omitting anything:

Fig. 7.10 Findings on general inspection of the abdomen in renal disease

Test	Sign	Diagnostic inference
look for abnormality of the abdominal contours: • general distension	• general fullness and enlargement of the abdominal cavity • the skin of the abdomen is shiny and smooth	renal causes of a distended abdomen are: • fluid (ascites or CAPD fluid) other (non-renal) causes include: • fat • flatus • fetus • faeces (constipation)
• localized distension: observe to see if abdomen moves with or independently of respiration	symmetrical swelling	polycystic kidneys
	asymmetrical swelling	enlarged kidney; kidney transplant in the iliac regions
look for scars: note position on the abdomen and check round to the back following the ribs to the spine	midline scars	previous abdominal surgery
	iliac scars overlying a mass	kidney transplant
	lateral longitudinal scars extending around the back	nephrectomy scars
	note that old scars are white and pale and recent scars are purple–red in colour	

Note: CAPD, continuous ambulatory peritoneal dialysis

- Begin with gentle palpation of the nine regions of the abdomen; then repeat using deeper palpation – keep looking at the patient's face for any signs of discomfort.
- Feel for the liver and spleen while the patient is breathing deeply in and out.
- Next examine the kidneys and urinary bladder, feeling for the aorta, and then check the hernial orifices (inguinal and femoral) while the patient is coughing.
- If you feel a mass, define its site, size, shape, edge, surface (regular or irregular), consistency, mobility, movement with respiration and whether it is pulsatile or resonant to percussion. Also check for associated scars and listen over the mass for a bruit.
- Remember to tell the patient that you need to examine the genitalia and to perform a digital rectal examination (see p. 153).

Figure 7.11 explains how the kidneys are examined and gives the relevant findings in various renal conditions. The differentiating features between an enlarged left kidney and splenomegaly are summarized in Figure 7.12.

The kidneys are usually not palpable except in very thin people. When they are enlarged, however, be careful, because an enlarged kidney can easily be confused with:

- Hepatomegaly (right)
- Splenomegaly (left).

Percussion

Percussion in the abdomen is used to elicit the cause of any distension and the composition of any mass – fluid-filled cysts and solid tumours are dull on percussion. Figure 7.13 shows the findings observed on percussion of the abdomen in patients with renal disease.

Remember the causes of a distended abdomen as the '5 Fs':

- Fat
- Fluid
- Flatus
- Fetus
- Faeces.

Fig. 7.11 How to examine the kidneys and relevant findings in a variety of renal conditions

Test	Sign	Diagnostic inference
bimanual examination of the kidneys (balloting): • place the right hand anteriorly in the lumbar region and the left hand posteriorly under the patient in the loin • push up with the left hand as the patient takes a deep breath • ballot the kidneys between both hands (i.e. push the kidney from one hand to the other) • repeat on the other side keeping the right hand anterior	the kidney is normally impalpable (except in very thin people) and if easily felt suggests an abnormality the lower pole is felt as a firm round edge between both hands on deep inspiration (it must be distinguished from an enlarged liver or spleen) there is minimal movement on respiration an irregular kidney surface felt in polycystic disease	unilateral enlargement: • tumour • renal cyst • hydronephrosis • compensatory hypertrophy bilateral enlargement: • polycystic kidneys • hydronephrosis • tumour (rare)
examination of the urinary bladder: • the bladder is palpated from the umbilicus down to the symphysis pubis • the upper and lateral borders are easily felt • the inferior border is impalpable	not normally palpable when enlarged it is felt as a smooth rounded firm cystic mass in the suprabupic region it is not always symmetrical and in the midline	chronic retention of urine accute retention is associated with bladder tenderness distended bladders are not always palpable in obesity
pain: • check carefully if the patient is in pain • the nature of the pain is important in determining the site of the lesion • assess pain by asking the patient to point to the pain and asking what the pain is like	fixed constant pain; colicky pain superimposed on a constant dull pain	kidney pain
	radiation of pain from the flank to the groin and iliac fossa; the patient is usually writhing in pain and is doubled up	ureteric distension due to obstruction in the ureters, most commonly renal stones as they are passed down the ureter

Fig. 7.12 Features that distinguish between left kidney enlargement and splenomegaly

Enlarged left kidney	Splenomegaly
moves late with inspiration	moves early in inspiration
can feel above it	cannot get above it; enlarges towards the umbilicus
smooth surface	notched border palpable
resonant to percussion	dull to percussion

Auscultation

Auscultate for bruits by applying the stethoscope firmly on the abdomen or in the flank over the renal artery. Alternatively, they can be heard over the back. However, it can be difficult to distinguish an aortic bruit from one originating in the renal artery. A bruit is heard if there is rapid turbulent movement of blood through a narrowed artery. Causes of bruits include:

- Renal artery stenosis
- Atherosclerosis
- Arteriovenous malformation in the kidney.

Digital rectal examination

Always obtain permission and have a chaperone for female patients. The patient should lie on the left side, with the knees drawn up to the chest.

Fig. 7.13 Findings on percussion of the abdomen in renal disease

Test	Sign	Diagnostic inference
ascites (excess free fluid in the peritoneal cavity): • presence shown by shifting of dullness • the abdomen is percussed from the flank into the midline for any areas of dullness • keep your hand on the area of dullness • ask the patient to roll away from you on to his or her side • percuss in this area with the patient in the new position and see if it is now resonant to percussion • this can be confirmed by asking the patient to roll over onto the other side	positive shifting dullness is indicative of ascites the area that was previously dull to percussion becomes resonant due to redistribution of fluid in the peritoneal cavity	causes of ascites in renal disease: • nephrotic syndrome • peritoneal dialysis • idiopathic ascites of dialysis • peritoneal dialysis fluid
percussion of the bladder: always percuss from above the umbilicus down to the pubic bone	resonance followed by dullness consistent with an enlarged cystic mass	distension of the urinary bladder due to chronic or acute retention

Fig. 7.14 Changes of the prostate noted on digital rectal examination

Sign	Diagnostic inference
firm, smooth, rubbery consistency; walnut shaped and sized	normal prostate
tender, enlarged and soft	acute infection (prostatitis)
hard, irregular, asymmetric, nodular	prostate carcinoma

- Inspect the perianal area for haemorrhoids, fissures, inflammation, prolapse and ulcers
- Put lubricant on the glove and insert finger into the rectum
- Assess the tone of the anal sphincter and the size and shape of the prostate (normally walnut sized)
- After removing your finger, inspect for any blood or faeces
- Feel for any lateral masses.

Palpable changes in the prostate and their clinical significance are summarized in Figure 7.14. A vaginal examination should also be performed in female patients. (See *Crash Course: Obstetrics and Gynaecology* for further details.)

Objectives

By the end of this chapter you should be able to:

- Name five tests that can be performed on a urine sample, and explain the importance of a mid-stream urine sample
- List the blood tests that can be done to investigate renal function, and give the possible causes of abnormal results
- Explain why plasma creatinine is a poor indicator of renal function
- Explain when you would use ultrasonography in preference to plain radiography
- List the indications and contraindications for a renal biopsy, and four potential complications
- Describe the complications of using intravenous contrast medium
- Explain the main differences between a diagnostic and a therapeutic cystoscopy
- Name the main investigation used to stage renal tumours
- Explain how urodynamics studies can be used to differentiate between genuine stress incontinence and urge incontinence.

Introduction

When considering investigations, always start with the least invasive simple procedures and then progress to second-line investigations if required.

TESTING THE BLOOD AND URINE

Diseases of the renal and urinary tract are suggested by symptoms linked to the urinary tract, abnormal urinalysis or abnormal serum urea or creatinine concentration. Testing the urine is the simplest investigation and should always be done in suspected renal disease. This is done with a mid-stream urine (MSU) sample, and assessment includes appearance, pH, dipstick, microscopy and cytological examination (Figs 8.1 and 8.2).

To take an MSU:

- The patient must have a full bladder
- Clean the external urethral meatus with a sterile swab
- Collect the sample half way through urine flow.

Plasma urea and creatinine are used to assess renal function. However, a significant amount of renal damage can occur before abnormal values are detected in the blood. The preferred option to assess renal function is the calculation of estimated glomerular filtration rate (eGFR) which closely reflects true GFR especially at the lower (clinically significant) end of the range (see Chapter 1). A full blood count may show anaemia (due to blood loss or impaired renal function). Other important blood results are shown in Figure 8.3.

IMAGING AND OTHER INVESTIGATIONS

Imaging is a very useful investigation in renal disease when used in conjunction with other investigative techniques. Radiological imaging of the upper and lower urinary tract can be used to:

- Establish a diagnosis
- Assess the complications of impaired renal function
- Monitor the progression of disease
- Follow the response to treatment.

Fig. 8.1 Microbiological tests and their significance

	Indications	Scientific basis	Normal results	Abnormal results
urine culture	must always be performed if UTI symptoms or any renal disease is suspected; in cases of TB an early morning sample of urine is required	growing any organisms present; vital to have an MSU specimen	no growth	>100 000 CFU/mL indicates urinary infection; <10 000 CFU/mL probably indicates contamination of the specimen
antibodies (i) streptococcal Ag	suspicion of past streptococcal glomerulonephritis	antibodies are made in response to infection and may trigger glomerulonephritis		increased titres of: anti-DNAase B ASOT consistent with poststreptococcal glomerulonephritis
(ii) hepatitis	renal disease associated with liver disease	infection with hepatitis B and C has effects on the kidney		hepatitis B causes: polyarteritis nodosa; membranous nephropathy hepatitis C causes: cryoglobulinaemia
(iii) HIV	patients at risk of HIV with renal symptoms	infection with HIV can cause renal damage		HIV-associated glomerulonephritis
malaria	those who have recently returned from the tropics and have recurrent fevers			ring-form parasites observed on peripheral blood film

Note: Ag, antigen; ASOT, antistreptococcal O antigen titre; CFU, colony-forming units; HIV, human immunodeficiency virus; MSU, mid-stream urine; TB, tuberculosis; UTI, urinary tract infection

- Imaging of the upper urinary tract includes KUB radiography, ultrasonography, CT, MRI and IVU.
- The main form of imaging for the lower urinary tract is cystoscopy.

The main type of radiograph used to visualize the renal system and urinary tract is a KUB, NOT a plain abdominal view, as this often does not include the full pelvis.

Plain radiography

Plain radiography of the kidney, ureters and bladder (KUB) is a simple, non-invasive test that can be used before specialized imaging. It is used to detect calcification in the kidney, such as renal and urinary tract stones – uric acid stones cannot be detected, but in general 90% of stones are radio-opaque (Figs 8.4 and 8.5). It also shows the size and position of the kidneys (this is unreliable), and any secondary bony deposits (such as can be associated with prostatic cancer).

Ultrasonography

Ultrasonography is a non-invasive technique that involves high frequency sound waves. It can accurately assess the size, shape and position of the kidney, and can also distinguish solid masses and renal cysts (Figs 8.6 and 8.7). Dilatation of the pelvicalyceal system and upper ureters can also be detected – suggesting the presence of urinary tract obstruction. This is a major cause of reversible renal failure, and can be treated if detected early enough. Transrectal ultrasound (TRUS) can also assess prostate size and

Fig. 8.2 Urine test results and their significance

	Indications	Scientific basis	Normal results	Abnormal results
appearance	any urine sample		clear fluid	**red/pink:** haematuria, beetroot intake **brown:** concentrated cholestatic jaundice **cloudy:** infection
volume	any urine sample		1000–2500 mL/day	**oliguria:** physiological; intrinsic renal disease; obstructive nephropathy **polyuria:** excess H_2O intake; increased solute loss e.g. glucose; concentration failure
pH	any urine sample		pH 4.5–8.0	**alkaline urine:** infection with *Proteus*–urea splitting **acid urine:** aminoaciduria; renal calculi
sodium	oliguria altered Na^+ homeostasis	urinary [Na] must be interpreted in context of urine output, sodium intake and natriuretic drugs	depends on clinical setting; 24-hour urinary Na^+ = 100–250 mmol/L	<20 mmol/L oliguria aminoaciduria; renal calculi <20 mmol/L oliguria →prerenal <20 mmol/L and not oliguric →extrarenal losses >20 mmol/L renal losses
creatinine and creatinine clearance	similar to those for blood creatinine levels	creatinine clearance reflects GFR; both the urine and plasma concentration of creatinine is required; requires timed urine collection	125 mL/min per 1.73 m^2 body surface area	decreased levels indicate a decrease in GFR—as seen in acute and chronic renal diseases
blood	gross bleeding into urine usually found in patients with renal disease; hypertension; pregnancy; bacterial endocarditis	reagent strips are used – based on a peroxide-like reaction	nil any positive result must be followed by microscopy	**microscopic haematuria:** renal disease, i.e. nephritic syndrome; blood at the beginning of voiding then clear – from the urethra; blood throughout voiding – from the bladder or above; blood only at the end of voiding – from the prostate or base of the bladder
protein dipstick and if positive → protein or albumin to creatinine ratio (or 24-hour collection)	oedema	reagent strips impregnated with buffered blue tetrabromophenol – detects [albumin] >150 mg/L; microalbuminuria is used as an earlier indicator of diabetic glomerular disease; the test requires a radioimmunoassay ↑ which is more sensitive than the strips	PCR <45mg/mmol or <150 mg/day (>0.3g/L is detected on the sticks) microalbuminuria = 0.2–2.8 mg/mmol of creatinine or 30–150 µg/min	**increased with:** exercise; standing up; renal disease; nephrotic syndrome; fever; diabetic glomerular disease; hypertension
glucose	suspected diabetes mellitus; renal disease; pregnancy	reagent strips using glucose oxidase or hexokinase enzyme reactions Clinitest	nil	**glucose may be present when:** 1. blood glucose above the renal threshold i.e. diabetes mellitus 2. altered renal threshold i.e. pregnancy; renal disease
urine microscopy (obtain a clean urine sample i.e. MSU) **(i) direct** **(ii) after centrifugation**	symptoms of UTIs; suspicion of renal disease	a small amount of unspun urine placed on a slide, covered with a cover slip and looked at under a microscope Gram stain to look for bacteria counterstained to look at cytology	nil	**white cells indicate:** inflammatory reaction; infection in the urinary tract; stones; TB; analgesic nephropathy **red cells indicate:** glomerulonephritis; acute urinary tract infection; calculi; tumour **granular casts indicate:** acute tubular necrosis; rapidly progressing glomerulonephritis **white blood cell casts indicate:** pyelonephritis **red cell casts indicate:** glomerulonephritis **crystals seen indicate:** stones **bacteria seen indicate:** infection **abnormal cells indicate:** cancer of urothelium

Note: MSU, mid-stream urine; TB tuberculosis; UTI, urinary tract infection; GFR, glomerular filtration rate; PCR, polymerase chain reaction

Fig. 8.3 Blood test results and their significance

	Indications	Scientific basis	Normal results	Abnormal results
urea	oliguria & anuria; dehydration; hypertension; diabetes mellitus; oedema; nausea and vomiting; loin pain	crude indication of renal function	2.5–6.6 mmol/L	increased in: renal disease; high protein intake; fever; gastrointestinal haemorrhage
creatinine	same as above for urea	reciprocal relationship with GFR – reflects renal function	60–120 µmol/L	increased in all types of renal disease; N.B. GFR may fall by 50% before urea or creatinine go outside the reference range
albumin	oedema	gives an assessment of severity of urinary protein losses in proteinuria	35–50 g/L	hypoalbuminaemia nephrotic syndrome hyperalbuminaemia dehydration
sodium, potassium, anion gap	confusion; lethargy; seizures; coma; arrhythmias; hypertension; hypotension; tachycardia/ bradycardia; vomiting; diarrhoea; heavy sweating; diabetes mellitus; polyuria; polydipsia	changes in the concentration of sodium, potassium and the anion gap are found in renal diseases; potassium is important in the function of excitable tissues and is important for survival	Na = 135–145 mmol/L K = 3.5–5.0 mmol/L anion gap = 8–16 mmol/L	hypernatraemia hyponatraemia hyperkalaemia hypokalaemia increased anion gap in: renal failure ketoacidosis (diabetes mellitus) hyperlactaemia (from shock) anion ingestion
arterial blood gases and pH (uses arterial blood)	hypoperfusion; hyperventilation; Kussmaul's breathing in diabetic ketoacidosis; ingestion of acids; diarrhoea; vomiting	oxygen concentration is important as it reflects tissue perfusion; an increase in CO_2 is lethal and poisonous to cells; pH is vital because most cells in the body work at an optimal pH and are very sensitive to changes in pH	pO_2 = 10.6–13.0 kPa pCO_2 = 4.7–6.0 kPa pH = 7.35–7.45	acidosis commonly found in renal failure; compensated for by respiratory stimulation ↓ pCO_2
haemoglobin	chronic renal failure; haemorrhage	haemoglobin levels are important as it carries oxygen to the tissues	male 13.5–18.0 g/dL female 11.5–16.0 g/dL	decreased haemoglobin chronic renal failure blood loss polycythaemia renal tumours renal cysts
ESR	loin pain; symptoms of UTI; systemic disease		<15 mm/h	increased in: infection renal cell carcinoma retroperitoneal fibrosis vasculitis
PSA	any man aged >45 years with prostatism or UTI	the level of PSA increases with prostatic cancer and metastatic disease; used to monitor therapy success		increased in: prostatic carcinoma silent recurrence of carcinoma metastatic disease small increase in prostatic hyperplasia
urate	kidney stones; patients with large tumour loads given chemotherapy; 'tumour lysis' syndrome → urate	hyperuricaemia can cause urate deposition in renal tract	0.12–0.42 mmol/L	increased in: gout renal and urinary calculi
calcium	kidney stones; myeloma; metastatic disease	hypercalcaemia causes calcium deposition in renal tract; hypercalcuria also causes urinary concentrating defects	2.0–2.6 mmol/L	increased in: renal and urinary calculi
eGFR	monitoring known CKD, diabetes mellitus, hypertension, ACEi use	estimates renal function from creatinine using MDRD formula, allowing for differences in muscle mass resulting from age, sex and race	>90 mL/min/1.73m^2	decreased in renal failure

Note: UTI, urinary tract infection; GFR, glomerular filtration rate; PSA, prostate-specific antigen eGFR, estimated glomerular filtration rate; ESR, erythrocyte sedimentation rate; CKD, chronic kidney disease; ACEi, angiotensin-converting enzyme inhibitor. *MDRD, Modification of Diet in Renal Disease

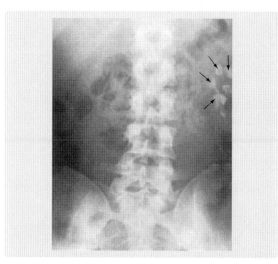

Fig. 8.4 Plain abdominal radiograph showing several calculi in the left kidney (arrows) (courtesy of Mr RS Cole).

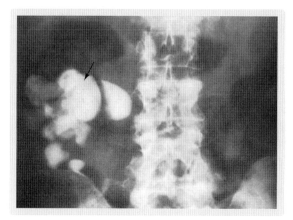

Fig. 8.5 This plain abdominal radiograph shows a large staghorn calculus (arrow) in the right kidney in a patient who presented with recurrent urinary tract infections (from Williams G, Mallick NP 1994 Color atlas of renal diseases, 2nd edn. Mosby Year Book).

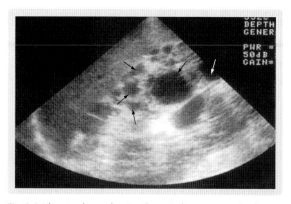

Fig. 8.6 Ultrasound scan showing the typical appearance of polycystic kidneys. There are multiple cysts (arrows) in the parenchyma (from Lloyd-Davis RW et al 1994 Color atlas of urology, 2nd edn. Mosby Year Book).

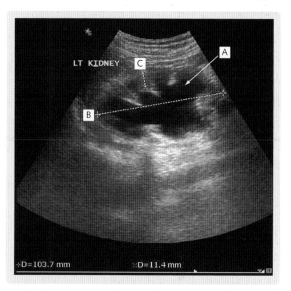

Fig. 8.7 Hydronephrosis of the left kidney demonstrated by ultrasonography. The echolucent (black) areas within the kidney are caused by dilated calyces (A). The bipolar length (B) of the kidney is normal and the cortical thickness (C) is well preserved, suggesting that prompt relief of the obstruction will allow good functional recovery.

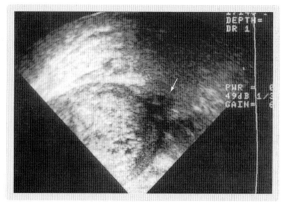

Fig. 8.8 A rectal ultrasound probe is used to define and stage carcinoma of the prostate. The arrow highlights an echo-poor area in the left peripheral zone of the prostate. This extends into the central part of the gland and beyond the capsule (courtesy of Dr D Rickards).

if necessary, be used to guide a prostate biopsy (Fig. 8.8). Renal vein thrombosis can be detected with Doppler ultrasonography, and arterial Doppler studies can be used to identify renal artery stenosis. The specificity and sensitivity of ultrasound investigations are very operator dependent.

Computed tomography

Computed tomography (CT) is a quick and non-invasive technique, which can be used with or

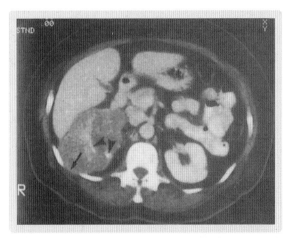

Fig. 8.9 CT scan highlighting a right renal cell carcinoma that extends through the intercostal space between ribs 11 and 12 (arrow) and medially along the renal vein. The high density (white) areas (arrows) indicate calcification (from Williams G, Mallick NP 1994 Color atlas of renal diseases, 2nd edn. Mosby Year Book).

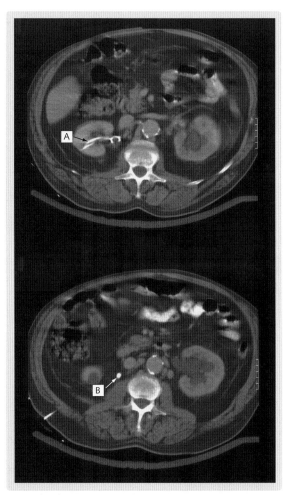

Fig. 8.10 An abdominal CT scan of a patient who presented with acute renal failure and bilateral loin pain. There is bilateral hydronephrosis secondary to bilateral ureteric stones. In the upper image a nephrostomy tube is seen in the right renal pelvis (A). The lower image demonstrates a dense opacity (calculus) lying in the ureter approximately at the level of L2 (B). Subsequent images demonstrated a similar opacity at L3 on the left.

without contrast. It is used to define renal and retroperitoneal masses and is ideal for locating and staging renal tumours (Fig. 8.9). It is also used to show polycystic kidney disease and has the advantage of also highlighting non-renal pathology. Modern techniques involving spiral CT can be used to visualize the anatomy of the renal arteries, renal vein and inferior vena cava, as well as retroperitoneal studies. Increasingly, CT is the investigation of choice to diagnose obstruction to the urinary tract (Fig. 8.10).

Renal biopsy

Renal biopsy is necessary to classify glomerulonephritis, which can influence the choice of therapy in patients with nephrotic syndrome and acute nephritis. It is also used in the diagnosis and assessment of systemic diseases that affect the kidneys, e.g. sarcoidosis and systemic lupus erythematosus. It can aid the investigation of unexplained acute renal failure, proteinuria, and haematuria and is vital in the management of patients with renal transplants. A sample of the kidney tissue can be taken by inserting a biopsy needle into the kidney under ultrasound guidance, with the patient lying in the prone position. This is then examined under a microscope, using immunochemical staining to detect complement or immunoglobulins. Relative contraindications to renal biopsy include:

- A bleeding diathesis (absolute unless corrected)
- Single kidney (risk of loss)
- Obesity (technically difficult)
- Small kidneys (technically difficult)
- Pregnancy
- Renal failure (increased risk of bleeding).

The main complications are pain, bleeding (haematuria or perinephric haematoma) or infection (rare).

Cystoscopy

A rigid or flexible cystoscope is inserted through the urethra to inspect the interior surface of the lower

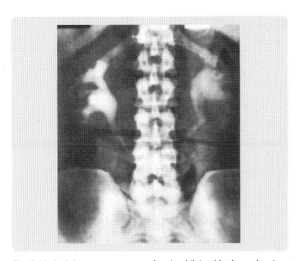

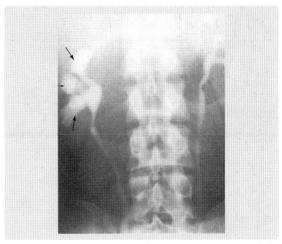

Fig. 8.11 An intravenous urogram showing bilateral hydronephrosis in response to bladder neck obstruction caused by dense granulation and fibrous tissue in a patient with schistosomiasis of the bladder (from Williams G, Mallick NP 1994 Color atlas of renal diseases, 2nd edn. Mosby Year Book).

Fig. 8.12 An intravenous urogram showing marked calyceal clubbing in the right kidney (arrows). There is gross dilatation of the calyces, which is pronounced in all poles of the kidney. These findings are the result of unilateral reflux of urine and chronic infection (from Lloyd-Davis RW et al 1994 Color atlas of urology, 2nd edn. Mosby Year Book).

urinary tract (bladder and urethra). This technique is very useful in the diagnosis and treatment of tumours in the bladder. It can also be used to identify stones and fistulae, take a tissue biopsy and to assess prostatic disease.

Diagnostic cystoscopy can be carried out in the outpatient clinic, and involves a flexible cystoscope examination under local anaesthesia. Therapeutic cystoscopy may require a hospital admission and uses a rigid cystoscope, with the patient under general anaesthesia.

Intravenous urography and intravenous pyelography

Intravenous urography (IVU) and pyelography (IVP) involve serial radiographs taken after intravenous injection of radio-opaque contrast medium (Figs 8.11 and 8.12). Normal kidney function is required, and the patient must not be pregnant. An IVU can assess kidney size and shape as well as the anatomy and patency of the calyces, pelvis and ureters. It can also be used to localize fistulae and highlight filling defects in the bladder.

Investigations involving contrast involve the risks of allergy to the contrast medium and renal damage (especially if there is pre-existing chronic kidney disease). Allergy can range from mild (itching, nausea and vomiting) to severe life-threatening anaphylaxis.

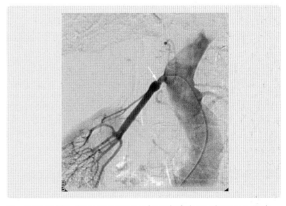

Fig. 8.13 Subtraction arteriogram of a right kidney. There is a single right renal artery with a significant stenosis at the ostium (arrow) with post-stenotic dilatation.

Previous reactions to contrast are a contraindication to its further use.

Renal arteriography

Conventional renal arteriography uses contrast medium to demonstrate the anatomy of the renal arteries. It is used to detect renal artery stenosis or aneurysms (Fig. 8.13). Therapeutic angioplasty may be performed at the same time. It can also be used in the diagnosis of tumours, but this is becoming less common with the increasing use of CT. A catheter is introduced into the femoral artery,

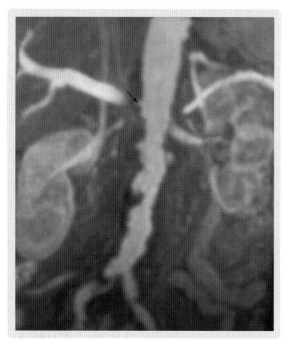

Fig. 8.14 Magnetic resonance renal angiography demonstrating a tight stenosis at the origin of the right renal artery (arrow). The irregularity of the abdominal aorta is due to marked atheroma.

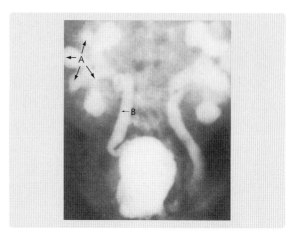

Fig. 8.15 A micturating cystourethrogram showing bilateral ureteric reflux. This patient has early calyceal clubbing (A) and ureteric dilatation (B). This is grade 3 reflux (courtesy of Mr RS Cole).

through which contrast is injected into the renal artery and a series of radiographs are taken.

Renal artery stenosis can also be detected using magnetic resonance imaging avoiding the use of potentially nephrotoxic contrast (Fig. 8.14).

Micturating cystourethrography

Micturating cystourethrograms are used to demonstrate vesicoureteric reflux from the bladder to the ureters during emptying of the bladder (Fig. 8.15). Reflux can be classified into three grades.

- Grade 1: contrast medium enters the ureter only
- Grade 2: contrast medium fills the pelvicalyceal system
- Grade 3: dilatation of the calyces and ureter.

This technique was used to investigate patients with recurrent urinary tract infections but has largely been replaced by other techniques because of concerns over ionizing radiation (especially in children).

Urodynamic studies

These are used to distinguish urge incontinence from genuine stress incontinence. They also detect

bladder/detrusor muscle instability. The bladder is catheterized and a pressure probe is inserted to measure the bladder pressure. A rectal probe is also inserted to assess intra-abdominal pressure. The detrusor muscle pressure can be calculated by subtracting the bladder pressure from the intra-abdominal pressure. The bladder is then filled with water until the patient feels the urge to void. At this point the relative pressures are recorded. If the patient has stress incontinence, an increase in intra-abdominal pressure (e.g. coughing) leads to involuntary urine leakage, with no bladder/detrusor muscle contraction. If the patient has urge incontinence, the bladder/detrusor muscle contracts either spontaneously or with increased abdominal pressure, and the patient feels an overwhelming urge to urinate immediately (Fig. 8.16).

Retrograde pyelography

Retrograde pyelography is used to define the site of an obstruction (Fig. 8.17) or lesions within the ureter. It does not require functioning kidneys. Under general anaesthesia a ureteric catheter is inserted into the ureter under cystoscopic guidance. Contrast medium is injected into the catheter to identify any lesions. It may be used therapeutically to help dislodge ureteric stones and coax them down the ureter.

Antegrade pyelography

This is used to define the site of obstruction in the upper urinary tract, i.e. mainly within the

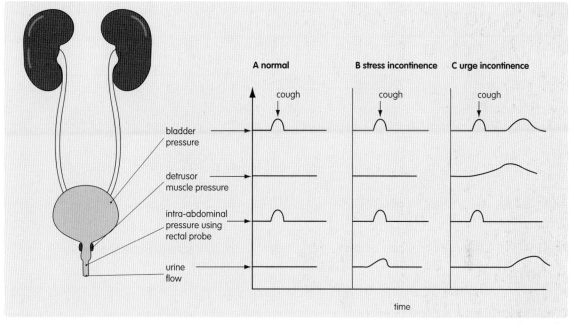

Fig. 8.16 Diagnosing incontinence using urodynamic studies. (A) Normal cough; (B) identifies stress incontinence, in which urine leakage is seen in response to raised intra-abdominal pressure; (C) shows urge incontinence, in which urine leakage is seen in response to detrusor muscle instability following a rise in intra-abdominal pressure.

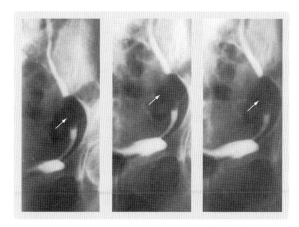

Fig. 8.17 Retrograde pyelogram showing a large filling defect in the left ureter (arrow) caused by a tumour (from Lloyd-Davis RW et al 1994 Color atlas of urology, 2nd edn. Mosby Year Book).

pelvicalyceal system. Following percutaneous catheterization of a renal calyx contrast medium is injected as described above for retrograde pyelography. Percutaneous catheterization of the pelvicalyceal system (nephrostomy) is also used therapeutically to relieve obstruction.

Magnetic resonance imaging

Magnetic resonance imaging (MRI) is an imaging technique that does not involve ionizing radiation – unlike CT. Instead, it relies on the measurement of the magnetic fields of atomic nuclei. It can differentiate cystic and solid renal masses and is useful for precise staging of tumours. However, MRI cannot be used in patients with pacemakers or other metallic implants. Magnetic resonance has now been developed to provide resolution sufficient to diagnose atheromatous renal artery stenosis (see Fig. 8.14).

Radionuclide scanning

Technetium-labelled dimercaptosuccinic acid (^{99m}Tc-DMSA) provides static images of the renal parenchyma. It highlights the localization, shape and function of each individual kidney, and highlights scarring as a result of reflux nephropathy (Fig. 8.18). Technetium-labelled pentetic acid (^{99m}Tc-DTPA) is excreted by renal filtration and the changes in the level of ^{99m}Tc-DTPA in the kidney over time are quantified using a gamma camera.

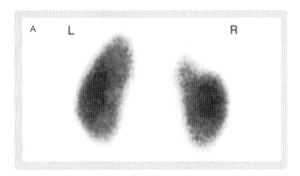

This provides a dynamic index of blood flow to each kidney. It is used to assess transplant function (Fig. 8.19A) and can demonstrate obstruction to the upper urinary tract (by diuresis renogram, Fig. 8.18B). It can also be used to determine the relative function of each kidney. Both ^{99m}Tc-DMSA and ^{99m}Tc-DTPA are injected into the venous circulation. Radionuclide techniques can be used to demonstrate reflux nephropathy.

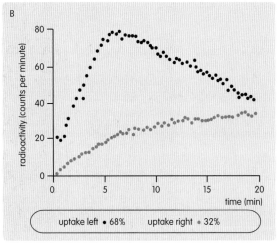

uptake left • 68%   uptake right • 32%

Fig. 8.18 (A) ^{99m}Tc-DMSA scan showing a right upper pole scar (courtesy of Dr TO Nunan). (B) The graph shows a diminished uptake of 36% for the right kidney, indicating a degree of loss of function correlating with the scar (from Williams G, Mallick NP 1994 Color atlas of renal diseases, 2nd edn. Mosby Year Book).

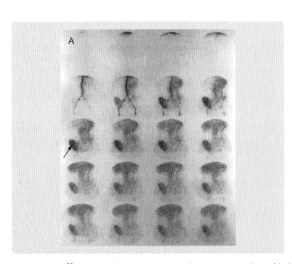

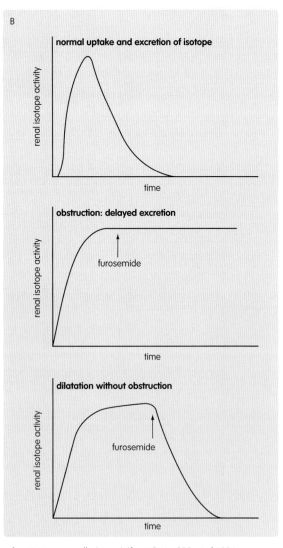

Fig. 8.19 (A) ^{99m}Tc-DTPA diuretic renogram showing a transplanted kidney functioning normally (arrow) (from Catto GRD et al 1994 Diagnostic picture tests in renal disease. TMIP). (B) Diuretic isotopic renography showing tracings for normal, obstructed and dilated (without obstruction) upper urinary tract. Obstruction can be distinguished from dilatation by administering furosemide, which promotes excretion of the isotope in dilatation (without obstruction) but has no effect on excretion rates in obstruction (from Johnson RJ, Feehally J 2000 Comprehensive nephrology. Mosby Year Book).

Other imaging techniques

Other imaging techniques include scintigraphy. This may be used to investigate vesicoureteric reflux in place of conventional imaging techniques, avoiding exposure to large doses of X-rays. Scintigraphy can also demonstrate secondary deposits in the bone (Fig. 8.20).

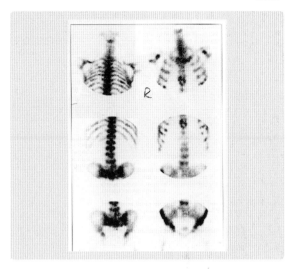

Fig. 8.20 This bone scintigram shows areas of increased activity in the ribs, sternum and pelvis (highlighted on the scan as dark 'hotspots'). This indicates multiple bone metastases in a patient with carcinoma of the prostate (courtesy of Dr TO Nunan).

SELF-ASSESSMENT

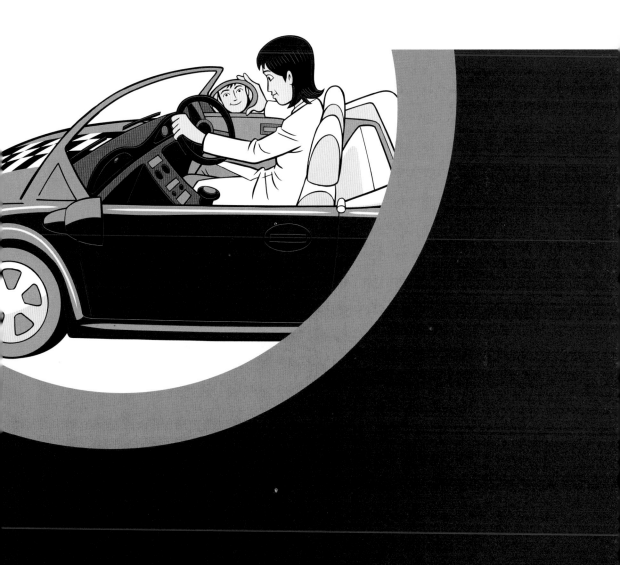

Indicate whether each answer is true or false.

Chapter 1 Basic principles

1. **Distribution of water:**
   a. Intracellular fluid (ICF) accounts for one-third of total body water (TBW).
   b. K is the major cation in ICF.
   c. Extracellular fluid (ECF) is composed of interstitial fluid, plasma and transcellular fluid.
   d. The major anions of ECF are Cl^- and HCO_3^-.
   e. Inulin is used to measure ICF.

2. **Subjects A and B are 70 kg males. Subject A drinks 2 L of distilled water and Subject B drinks 2 L of isotonic NaCl. As a result, subject B will have:**
   a. Greater change in ICF volume.
   b. Higher positive free water clearance.
   c. Greater change in plasma osmolarity.
   d. Higher urine osmolarity.
   e. Higher urine flow rate.

3. **Regarding fluid exchange between plasma and interstitial fluid (ISF):**
   a. Hydrostatic pressure at the arterial end of the capillary is 25 mmHg.
   b. Oncotic pressure varies along the capillary bed.
   c. Hydrostatic pressure is determined in part by arteriole blood pressure.
   d. Capillary membranes are permeable to plasma proteins.
   e. Fluid leaves plasma at the venous end of the capillary.

4. **Regarding the composition of fluid compartments:**
   a. There is a higher Cl^- concentration in the ICF than plasma.
   b. There are no proteins in the ECF.
   c. K^+ exists mostly extracellularly.
   d. Interstitial fluid is the same as transcellular fluid.
   e. Intracellular fluid makes up around 40% of our body weight.

5. **The following can be measured directly:**
   a. Total body water.
   b. Blood volume.
   c. Plasma volume.
   d. Intracellular volume.
   e. Interstitial fluid.

6. **Regarding water intake and output:**
   a. We lose per day 1500 mL of water from our skin and lungs.

   b. Water loss is increased in diarrhoea.
   c. Dehydration will result when total water intake in less than 1000 mL.
   d. The total amount of water lost should always exceed intake.
   e. Water only comes from food and drink.

7. **Osmoreceptors:**
   a. Detect variations in plasma osmolality.
   b. Are located in the thalamus.
   c. Receive blood supply from the internal carotid artery.
   d. Are the only stimulus for ADH release.
   e. Regulate the release of ADH.

Chapter 2 Organization of the kidneys ANATOMY

8. **Regarding the basic organization and function of the renal and urinary system:**
   a. The renal artery is a branch of the abdominal aorta.
   b. Urine is drained to the bladder from the kidney via the urethra, and from the bladder via the ureter.
   c. The urinary tract epithelium is permeable to water and solutes.
   d. Renin is produced by the macula densa cells in the juxtaglomerular apparatus (JGA).
   e. Bowman's capsule is located in the cortex of the kidney.

9. **Regarding the loop of Henle:**
   a. All nephrons have loops of Henle that enter the medulla.
   b. The thin descending loop is impermeable to water.
   c. The thin ascending loop is impermeable to water.
   d. The thick ascending loop transports sodium in the same way as the proximal tubule.
   e. ADH acts on the descending loop of Henle to increase its permeability to water.

10. **The right kidney:**
    a. Lies posterior to the second part of the duodenum.
    b. Lies immediately lateral to the aorta.
    c. Is higher than the left kidney.
    d. Lies anterior to psoas muscle.
    e. Has a colonic impression on its anterior surface.

Chapter 3 Renal function

11. The anion gap:

a. Is normally 20–25 mmol/L.
b. Is increased in renal tubular acidosis.
c. Is normal after salicylate ingestion.
d. Can be abnormal in chronic uraemia.
e. Is affected by lactic acidosis.

12. Thiazide diuretics:

a. Cause metabolic acidosis.
b. Cause hyperuricaemia.
c. Cause glucose intolerance.
d. Cause hypocalcaemia.
e. Are used in the treatment of angina.

13. A woman with a history of severe renal failure has the following arterial blood values:

pH 7.25, pCO_2 3.2 kPa, HCO_3^- 10 mmol/L. The correct diagnosis is:

a. Normal acid–base status.
b. Metabolic acidosis.
c. Metabolic alkalosis.
d. Respiratory acidosis.
e. Respiratory alkalosis.

14. Potassium excretion by the kidney varies according to:

a. The electrical profile of the distal nephron (i.e. degree of electronegativity of tubule lumen compared with that of blood).
b. Urine flow rate.
c. Urinary Na^+ concentration.
d. Plasma pH.
e. Plasma aldosterone concentration.

15. Control of glomerular filtration rate (GFR):

a. The tuboglomerular feedback mechanism responds to changes in arterial pressure.
b. The myogenic mechanism responds to changes in the composition of the tubular fluid.
c. The GFR is dependent on the renal blood flow (RBF).
d. Tubule NaCl concentrations affect GFR.
e. Detection of plasma protein concentration is vital to feedback control of GFR.

16. Match the following blood gas results with one of the clinical situations listed below: pH 7.3, pCO_2 6.8 kPa, pO_2 8.0 kPa:

a. Hyperventilation.
b. Diabetic ketoacidosis.
c. Pyloric stenosis.
d. Morphine.
e. High altitude.

17. Regarding the role of the proximal tubule in solute transport:

a. Glucose is transported by passive diffusion down its concentration gradient.
b. At plasma glucose levels of 10 mmol/L or above, glycosuria occurs.
c. A fall in GFR will result in a decreased plasma phosphate concentration.
d. Carbonic anhydrase plays an important role in HCO_3^- reabsorption.
e. K^+ secretion depends on aldosterone levels.

18. Regarding the counter current multiplier:

a. The role of the counter current multiplier is to produce a hypotonic medulla to concentrate urine.
b. The active reabsorption in the thick ascending limb ensures the osmolality of the interstitium is greater than that of the tubule.
c. Water is thus reabsorbed in the thick ascending limb.
d. NaCl moves into the filtrate in the descending limb.
e. At the tip of the loop the maximum osmolality of the interstitium is 600 mOsmol/kg H_2O.

19. Regarding secretion by the proximal tubule:

a. K^+ secretion is dependent on aldosterone levels.
b. H^+ secretion is independent of Na^+ transport.
c. Strong organic acids are gradient-time limited.
d. Acid–base status has no effect on K^+ secretion.
e. EDTA is a T_m-limited secretory mechanism.

20. Regarding glomerular filtration:

a. Negatively charged molecules are less readily filtered.
b. Filtration is driven by the oncotic pressure from the tubular fluid.
c. The basement membrane lies between the podocytes and glomerular endothelial cells.
d. Diabetes has no effect on glomerular filtration.
e. Normal glomerular filtrate contains large amounts of protein.

21. Regarding measurement of the GFR:

a. Creatinine may be used.
b. Clearance ratios compare the clearance of a substance with p-aminohippurate (PAH).
c. The estimated GFR (eGFR) is calculated using the clearance equation.
d. The eGFR may be used in the classification of chronic kidney disease.
e. Inulin is an endogenous molecule.

22. Match the following blood gas results with one of the clinical situations listed below: pH 7.5, pCO_2 3.7 kPa, pO_2 14.4 kPa:

a. Hyperventilation.
b. Diabetic ketoacidosis.
c. Pyloric stenosis.
d. Mild asthma.
e. COPD.

23. Regarding renal blood flow:

a. RBF is constant over a wide range of systemic arterial blood pressure.

b. PAH is used to measure RBF because it is reabsorbed by the proximal tubule.
c. The myogenic mechanism is the sole autoregulation system responsible for maintaining a constant RBF and GFR.
d. Vasoconstriction of the afferent arteriole leads to an increase in RBF.
e. Adenosine and nitric oxide have opposite effects on RBF.

24. **Match the following blood gas results with one of the clinical situations listed below: pH 7.34, pCO_2 7.3 kPa, pO_2 8.8 kPa**

a. Hyperventilation.
b. Diabetic ketoacidosis.
c. Pyloric stenosis.
d. Antacid ingestion.
e. Chronic obstructive pulmonary disease.

25. **Regarding antidiuretic hormone (ADH or vasopressin):**

a. Osmoreceptors are found in the thalamus in the brain.
b. It is released when thirsty.
c. Aquaporin 2 (AQP2) channels are activated by the binding of ADH to a V2 receptor on the basolateral membrane.
d. Alcohol may increase ADH release.
e. ADH results in a decrease in collecting duct permeability.

26. **Regarding problems of osmotic regulation:**

a. Polyuria and polydipsia are both symptoms of syndrome of inappropriate ADH secretion (SIADH).
b. Plasma ADH levels are normal in nephrogenic diabetes insipidus.
c. Polycystic kidneys may be a cause of neurogenic diabetes insipidus.
d. CNS or lung diseases may be a cause of SIADH.
e. Hyponatraemia is a sign of SIADH.

27. **The following statements are correct:**

a. The kidneys receive approximately 20% of the cardiac output.
b. In healthy young adults approximately 120 mL/min of protein-free filtrate is formed in the glomerulus.
c. Non-protein-bound drugs of molecular weight less than 66 kDa pass into the filtrate.
d. Potentially saturable mechanisms for active secretion of both acids and bases exist in the proximal tubule.
e. Low lipid solubility favours tubular reabsorption.

28. **Low renin levels are associated with:**

a. Hypoaldosteronism.
b. Addison's disease.
c. A decrease in potassium intake.
d. A rise in ECF volume.
e. A fall in plasma Na^+.

29. **Regarding regulation of calcium and phosphate:**

a. Parathyroid hormone (PTH) is released in response to a rise in plasma Ca^{2+}.
b. PTH release causes a decrease in urinary phosphate.
c. 70% of all plasma Ca^{2+} is reabsorbed in the proximal tubule.
d. Alkalosis is a cause of hypocalcaemia.
e. Renal calculi are a sign of hypocalcaemia.

30. **Regarding plasma potassium levels:**

a. Hyperkalaemia can be life threatening.
b. Severe vomiting may cause hypokalaemia.
c. ADH has no effect on K^+ transport in the kidney.
d. Aldosterone increases potassium reabsorption.
e. Furosemide removes potassium from the body.

31. **The following would increase GFR:**

a. Hyperproteinaemia.
b. A ureteral stone.
c. Dilatation of the afferent arteriole.
d. Dilatation of the efferent arteriole.
e. Constriction of the efferent arteriole.

32. **Erythropoietin secretion can be increased by:**

a. Angiotensin-converting enzyme (ACE) inhibitors.
b. Hypoxia.
c. Renal cell carcinoma.
d. Loss of renal substance.
e. Nephrotic syndrome.

33. **Plasma creatinine concentration:**

a. Is unaffected by body habitus.
b. Is a sensitive guide to mild renal impairment.
c. May be affected by drugs.
d. Is disproportionately increased compared with urea in rhabdomyolysis.
e. Reflects glomerular filtration.

34. **The following are causes of metabolic acidosis:**

a. Vomiting.
b. Uncontrolled insulin-dependent diabetes mellitus.
c. Chronic renal failure.
d. Salicylate poisoning.
e. Hyperaldosteronism.

Chapter 4 The kidneys in disease

35. **Regarding problems with embryological renal development:**

a. Horseshoe kidney is more common in girls.
b. Stone formation can occur in hypoplastic kidneys.
c. The incidence of ectopic kidneys is 1 in 20.
d. Agenesis of the kidney occurs in Potter's syndrome.
e. The ureters of an ectopic kidney are normal.

36. Minimal glomerular disease:

a. Is the commonest cause of the nephrotic syndrome in children.
b. Is characterized by podocyte changes seen under the light microscope.
c. Is associated with increased risk of infection.
d. Is treated with antibiotics.
e. Has a better prognosis in adults.

37. Regarding polycystic kidney disease (PKD):

a. It may lead to renal failure.
b. It never affects children.
c. Onset in adults could be due to the presence of a PKD gene.
d. Renal function tests are abnormal.
e. The cysts are confined to the cortex of the kidney(s).

38. Membranoproliferative glomerulonephritis (GN):

a. Is usually secondary to systemic diseases such as systemic lupus erythematosus (SLE).
b. Often involves activation of the classical complement pathway.
c. Is commonly seen in men over the age of 40.
d. Can be asymptomatic.
e. Can recur following transplantation.

39. IgA nephropathy:

a. Presents with urinary tract infection (UTI).
b. Is most common in India.
c. Is associated with mesangial proliferation.
d. Can be cured.
e. Has a worse prognosis in patients with hypertension.

40. Regarding Goodpasture's syndrome:

a. It is characterized by glomerular basement membrane autoantibodies.
b. Patients present with 'crescentic' glomerulonephritis.
c. Renal function gradually deteriorates, resulting in chronic renal failure.
d. It is associated with lung haemorrhage.
e. It requires supportive treatment only.

41. Bacterial endocarditis:

a. Can present with haematuria.
b. Causes a cystic disease of the kidney.
c. With treatment of endocarditis, renal lesions resolve.
d. Renal function tests may be abnormal.
e. Causes immune complex deposition in the glomeruli.

42. Henoch–Schönlein purpura (HSP):

a. Occurs in adults only.
b. Can follow an upper respiratory tract infection.
c. Is an infective inflammatory condition.
d. May present with arthralgia.
e. Is associated with a glomerulonephritis.

43. Urinary tract infections:

a. Are common in pregnancy.
b. *Escherichia coli* is commonly responsible for community-acquired UTIs.
c. Diagnosis of UTI is made on the clinical presentation alone.
d. Are caused by chronic non-steroidal anti-inflammatory drug (NSAID) use.
e. Are rarely seen in people with diabetes.

44. Diabetic nephropathy:

a. Only occurs in insulin-dependent diabetes mellitus (IDDM).
b. Is rare before 20 years of age.
c. Can present as the nephrotic syndrome.
d. Once present, usually progresses to end-stage renal failure.
e. Is characterized by microhaematuria.

45. Renal cell carcinoma:

a. Most commonly presents with haematuria.
b. Is more common is men.
c. Does not metastasize.
d. May increase erythropoietin production.
e. Smoking is the sole known risk factor.

46. Factors which predispose to urinary calculi include:

a. Being female and under 40 years of age.
b. Dehydration.
c. Hypocalcaemia.
d. Thiazide diuretics.
e. Cushing's syndrome.

47. Life-threatening complications of acute glomerulonephritis include:

a. Hypertensive encephalopathy.
b. Pulmonary oedema.
c. Uraemia.
d. Thrombocytopenia.
e. Thrombotic stroke.

48. In a patient in shock:

a. Blood pressure will be high.
b. Peripheral vasoconstriction will be one of the compensatory mechanisms.
c. Prostaglandins and angiotensin II act synergistically to cause renal vasoconstriction.
d. Aldosterone levels increase.
e. Acid–base balance is *never* disturbed.

49. Typical renal causes of oedema include:

a. Acute GN.
b. Nephrotic syndrome.
c. Nephrogenic diabetes insipidus.
d. Bladder transitional cell carcinoma.
e. Cystitis.

50. Hypertension may be caused by:

a. Renal artery stenosis.
b. Unknown causes.
c. UTI.

d. Addison's disease.
e. Chronic GN.

51. ACE inhibitors:

a. Inhibit the conversion of renin to angiotensin II.
b. Relieve symptoms, and prolong life in congestive cardiac failure.
c. Are safe in pregnancy.
d. Can cause hyperkalaemia.
e. Reduce proteinuria in diabetic nephropathy.

52. Loop diuretics:

a. Are weak diuretics.
b. Reduce calcium excretion.
c. Act in the thin descending loop of Henle.
d. Relieve pulmonary oedema.
e. Can cause gynaecomastia.

53. Dialysis:

a. Is indicated in all stages of chronic kidney disease.
b. Can be performed by more than one method.
c. An arteriovenous fistula is the preferred form of vascular access.
d. Peritoneal dialysis has no known complications.
e. Haemodialysis has no known complications.

54. Renal transplantation:

a. Is the first-line treatment for acute renal failure.
b. Renal transplants, unlike other transplants carry no risk of rejection.
c. Is placed in the normal position of the kidneys.
d. Immunosuppression is vital following the operation.
e. Graft survival is better with a live donor than a cadaver.

55. Carbonic anhydrase inhibitors:

a. Cause oedema.
b. Enhance bicarbonate reabsorption.
c. May lead to metabolic acidosis.
d. Are strong diuretics.
e. Are only used in renal disease.

56. Polyarteritis nodosa (PAN) characteristically:

a. Is more common in females.
b. Presents in old age.
c. May present with constitutional symptoms such as fever and arthralgia.
d. Affects medium-sized arteries.
e. Is associated with aneurysms.

57. Wilms' tumour:

a. Usually affects adults.
b. Is usually unilateral.
c. Is usually benign.
d. Presents most commonly as a painless abdominal mass.
e. Long-term survival is over 80%.

58. Potter's syndrome:

a. Is associated with unilateral renal agenesis.
b. Involves pulmonary hypoplasia.
c. Is associated with polyhydramnios.
d. Is incompatible with life.
e. Clinical features include low-set ears and an underdeveloped mandible.

59. Vesicoureteric reflux:

a. Is always congenital.
b. Can result from an abnormal entry of the ureters into the bladder.
c. Usually resolves by adulthood.
d. Can lead to renal failure.
e. Is best diagnosed by cystoscopy.

60. Wegener's granulomatosis:

a. Usually presents by the age of 20.
b. Is a necrotizing vasculitis.
c. Is an inherited disease.
d. Characteristically presents with abdominal pain and a purpuric skin rash on the extensor surfaces.
e. Can be treated by cyclophosphamide.

61. Adrenocortical insufficiency:

a. Results in decreased osmolarity of ECF.
b. Results in increased ECF volume.
c. Results in increased haematocrit.
d. Can occur when exogenous corticosteroid administration is discontinued.
e. Results in hypokalaemia.

62. The following can be features of nephritic syndrome:

a. Oliguria.
b. Low blood pressure.
c. Haematuria.
d. Decreased serum urea and creatinine.
e. Evidence of a recent streptococcal infection.

Chapter 5 The lower urinary tract

63. Regarding the bladder:

a. The neck is very mobile.
b. The external urethral sphincter is under involuntary control.
c. It lies inferior to the prostate.
d. It receives both sympathetic and parasympathetic innervation.
e. Blood supply is from the gluteal arteries.

64. Benign prostatic hypertrophy (BPH):

a. Occurs most often in men under 60 years of age.
b. Is associated with median lobe enlargement.
c. Acute retention may require surgical treatment.
d. Can metastasize.
e. Can present with UTI.

65. **Bladder transitional cell carcinoma (TCC):**
    a. Is usually benign.
    b. Is associated with cigarette smoking.
    c. Has a higher incidence in Egypt.
    d. Presents with a painful haematuria.
    e. Usually occurs on the posterior and lateral walls of the bladder.

66. **The following may affect micturition:**
    a. Multiple sclerosis.
    b. Increases in sympathetic tone.
    c. Hypertension.
    d. Minor vomiting.
    e. Spina bifida.

67. **Regarding structural abnormalities of the urinary tract:**
    a. Bifid ureters have no clinical effects.
    b. Hypospadias is very common, occurring in about 1 in 10 of the population.
    c. Exstrophy, despite treatment, carries a risk of adenocarcinoma development in later life.
    d. Hydroureters are only congenital.
    e. Urethral valves rarely cause serious clinical problems.

68. **Which one of the following is *not* a cause of urinary tract obstruction?**
    a. Calculi.
    b. Congenital abnormalities.
    c. Pregnancy.
    d. Nephrotic syndrome.
    e. Prostatic carcinoma.

69. **Schistosomiasis:**
    a. Is the most common blood fluke infection in the UK.
    b. Presents commonly with recurrent haematuria.
    c. Settles in the liver and the kidneys.
    d. Can lead to cystitis.
    e. Requires conservative treatment only.

70. **Risk factors for pyelonephritis include:**
    a. Being male and under 40 years of age.
    b. Pregnancy.
    c. Diabetes mellitus.
    d. Vesicoureteric reflux.
    e. Previous urinary tract surgery.

71. **Regarding voluntary control of micturition:**
    a. Voiding is controlled by sympathetic innervation.
    b. The relaxation of the internal and external urethral sphincters occurs before the urge to urinate.
    c. In order to void urine, the bladder must relax.
    d. The internal urethral sphincter contains smooth muscle.
    e. Stretching of the bladder wall stimulates stretch receptors.

72. **Carcinoma of the prostate:**
    a. Is common is young men.
    b. Presents with prostatism.
    c. Is always confined within the prostate.
    d. The first investigation required is an ultrasound scan.
    e. Prognosis depends on the stage.

73. **The urethra:**
    a. Is longer in men than in women.
    b. In men, has the same structure throughout.
    c. In both men and women lymphatic drainage is into the deep inguinal lymph nodes.
    d. In women opens up into the posterior wall of the vagina.
    e. In men passes lateral to the prostate.

74. **Clinical features of urinary tract stones are:**
    a. Asymptomatic.
    b. Haematuria.
    c. Renal colic.
    d. UTI.
    e. Urinary tract obstruction.

75. **The following conditions can present with microscopic haematuria:**
    a. Diabetic nephropathy.
    b. Polyarteritis nodosa.
    c. Renal calculi.
    d. Amyloidosis.
    e. Heavy exercise.

76. **Regarding urinary casts:**
    a. Hyaline casts in urine are always pathological.
    b. The presence of up to five red blood cell casts in urine is normal.
    c. White cell casts are detected in acute pyelonephritis.
    d. Tubular cell casts are seen in acute tubular necrosis.
    e. Red cell casts are diagnostic of nephrotic syndrome.

Chapter 6 Common presentations of renal disease

77. **The following could cause proteinuria:**
    a. Ureteric calculi.
    b. Hypospadias.
    c. Minimal change glomerulonephritis.
    d. Diabetes.
    e. Malaria.

78. **Regarding hyperuricaemia:**
    a. It always causes gout.
    b. It may occur following chemotherapy.
    c. It may be caused by drugs.
    d. Haematuria may be a presenting symptom.
    e. Hyperuricaemia refers to excess urate levels in the urine.

79. Regarding disorders of serum potassium and sodium:

a. Hypernatraemia can occur in diabetes mellitus.
b. Hyponatraemia always indicates a high ECF volume.
c. Conn's syndrome may lead to hyperkalaemia.
d. Too much insulin in diabetic people increases plasma K^+.
e. Acid–base disturbances can affect K^+ balance.

80. Acute renal failure:

a. Can be caused by Wegener's granulomatosis.
b. Can be irreversible.
c. Is always associated with abnormalities on urine dipstick.
d. Is a recognized complication of NSAID use.
e. Can be treated effectively by dopamine infusion.

81. The following can impair renal function:

a. Naproxen.
b. Ranitidine.
c. Iodine-containing contrast media.
d. Captopril.
e. Amphotericin B.

82. Urethral discharge:

a. Is always caused by a sexually transmitted infection.
b. Blood tests are the only investigation necessary.
c. Can be associated with Reiter's syndrome.
d. The discharge is typically clear.
e. Asking about the sexual history is important.

83. Acute tubular necrosis:

a. Can present initially with oliguria.
b. Is often reversible.
c. Is associated with hypokalaemia.
d. Can be precipitated by sepsis.
e. Small kidneys are typically found on ultrasound scan.

84. Nephrotic syndrome can be caused by:

a. Gold.
b. Penicillamine.
c. Staphylococcal infection.
d. Captopril.
e. Paracetamol.

85. Renal calculi:

a. Are always asymptomatic.
b. May result from high plasma calcium levels.
c. Can occur in people with gout.
d. Can be caused by hypoparathyroidism.
e. Cannot be prevented.

86. Regarding urinary incontinence:

a. It can occur in women who have multiple pregancies
b. It can be caused by neurological problems.
c. Overflow incontinence is associated with an increase in intra-abdominal pressure.

d. Nocturnal enuresis can never be acquired.
e. It is important to exclude an infection in the first line of any investigations or interventions.

87. Predisposing factors in UTI are:

a. Vesicoureteric reflux.
b. Diabetes mellitus.
c. Postmenopausal state.
d. Neurogenic bladder.
e. Structural urinary tract abnormality.

88. Recurrent UTIs can be prevented by:

a. Voiding before and after sexual intercourse.
b. Voiding at regular 2–3-h intervals.
c. Adequate control of diabetes.
d. A 2 L daily intake of fluid.
e. Treatment with immunosuppressive drugs.

89. Membranous glomerulonephropathy:

a. Is characterized by basement membrane thickening.
b. Is more common in females.
c. A similar histological pattern is typically seen in Henoch-Schönlein purpura.
d. Usually presents acutely.
e. Can only be treated with renal replacement therapy.

90. Treatment with corticosteroids is beneficial in patients with GN caused by:

a. A streptococcal throat infection.
b. Polyarteritis nodosa.
c. Systemic lupus erythematosus.
d. Bacterial endocarditis.
e. Wegener's granulomatosis.

Chapter 7 History and examination

91. When taking a history in a patient with suspected renal disease, which of the following would be relevant to ask about?

a. Hypertension.
b. Haematuria.
c. Recent throat infection.
d. Recent travel.
e. Family history of diabetes.

92. In relation to renal disease:

a. There are no nail signs.
b. Conjunctiva may be pale in chronic kidney disease.
c. Oedema of the face is never due to a renal cause.
d. A dry cough may occur following treatment of hypertension.
e. Limb length discrepancies can only have an orthopaedic cause.

93. Regarding the examination of the abdomen:

a. The patient should be at 90 degrees.
b. Inspection is irrelevant.
c. Always approach from the left-hand side of the patient.
d. The signs of an enlarged left kidney and an enlarged spleen are identical.
e. Ascites only has gastrointestinal causes.

94. Regarding the examination of the prostate:

a. Prostate carcinoma feels smooth.
b. A soft prostate is a healthy prostate.
c. Feeling for the size of the prostate is not important.
d. Permission must be obtained.
e. Walnut-shaped describes a normal prostate.

Chapter 8 Investigation and imaging

95. Regarding renal imaging:

a. A 'kidney/ureter/bladder' (KUB) X-ray is the same as an abdominal X-ray.
b. Plain radiography always detects calculi.
c. A micturating cystogram is used to confirm vesicoureteric reflux.
d. CT is used to stage renal tumours.
e. Renal arteriography involves contrast injected into the renal vein.

96. Ultrasound is useful to investigate renal disease because it can:

a. Differentiate between solid and cystic masses.
b. Provide information about the functional capacity of each kidney.
c. Highlight the anatomy of the ureters.
d. Assess prostatic enlargement in males.
e. Always diagnose the cause of acute renal failure.

97. Regarding urine biochemistry:

a. The presence of nitrites is non-pathological.
b. Urine may be assessed with a dipstick.
c. The presence of ketones should prompt further investigation.
d. Red/pink urine may have non-pathological causes.
e. Glycosuria is only found in diabetes.

98. Regarding blood biochemistry:

a. Creatinine can be used to measure renal function accurately.
b. Raised level of prostrate-specific antigen (PSA) confirms prostate carcinoma.
c. Hypercalcaemia may be found in patients with urinary calculi.
d. The erythrocyte sedimentation rate (ESR) is a measure of inflammation.
e. Very high levels of arterial bicarbonate and normal levels of CO_2 indicate acidosis.

99. Renal biopsy:

a. Is required to allow the histological classification of GN.
b. Involves a needle being inserted into the anterior abdominal wall.
c. Is usually done under X-ray guidance.
d. Massive obesity is a relative contraindication.
e. Has no complications.

100. Regarding urine microscopy:

a. Red cell casts indicate glomerulonephritis.
b. Smooth, brown and soft crystals suggest calcium-containing stones.
c. Bacteria are normally found in healthy individuals.
d. Blood clots indicate the need for further investigation.
e. May be used to diagnose a UTI.

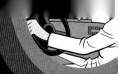

1. Describe the different fluid compartments within the body.

2. Describe the renal blood supply.

3. Explain the Gibbs–Donnan effect and how it is balanced.

4. Give two examples of how failure of the normal development of the renal tract can lead to anatomical abnormalities.

5. Write a short note on the structure of the nephron.

6. How are the renal blood flow and glomerular filtration rate regulated?

7. Describe the action of antidiuretic hormone on the collecting ducts.

8. Explain the role of renin in regulating body fluid volume.

9. Discuss the transport of glucose in the proximal tubule and how this relates to plasma glucose levels.

10. Describe the mechanisms underlying calcium and phosphate homeostasis.

11. Outline the systemic disorders which affect the glomerulus.

12. Summarize the effects of diabetes on the kidney.

13. Describe the TNM staging for transitional cell carcinoma of the bladder.

14. Write a short note on renal artery stenosis (RAS) and explain why angiotensin-converting enzyme (ACE) inhibitors are contraindicated in patients with RAS.

15. Discuss the complications resulting from abnormal blood potassium levels.

16. Write a short note on the complications of benign prostatic hypertrophy.

17. A 62-year-old known hypertensive patient presents with a left-sided stroke. Examination reveals a blood pressure of 173/100 mmHg, with xanthelasma and xanthoma. Bilateral corneal arcus is seen and bilateral abdominal bruits and a right-sided carotid bruit can be heard. Plasma creatinine is elevated at 240 µmol/L. Blood cholesterol is elevated.

   a. What is the significance of the bruits?
   b. What is the likely diagnosis?
   c. Which investigation would confirm this?
   d. Why are angiotensin-converting enzyme inhibitors contraindicated in this patient?
   e. Does the patient require dialysis?
   f. List three aspects of management.

18. A 74-year-old man presents with difficulty in starting micturition and a poor urinary stream with dribbling at the end of the stream. He also has nocturia, waking up six times a night to pass urine.

   a. What must be included in the clinical examination?
   b. What are the main differentials?
   c. What blood test can be performed to confirm the diagnosis?

19. A 7-year-old Asian boy presents with a 3-day history of oedema around the eyes, which is worse on waking. The parents report a reduced urine output, which appears 'frothy'. Examination reveals ankle and abdominal oedema, with reduced breath sounds (particularly on the right). There is also some scrotal swelling.

   a. What is the most likely diagnosis?
   b. List three useful investigations.
   c. Describe the management of this child.

20. A 35-year-old man presents with painful micturition. In particular, he finds the pain worse at the end of micturition, sometimes spreading to his penis. The pain is exacerbated by sudden movements, and is relieved by lying down. Over the past week, he has also noticed that the urine appears bloody towards the end of micturition.

   a. What is the most likely cause of the pain?
   b. Why is the pain referred to the penis, and why is it relieved on lying down?
   c. What is the investigation of choice to confirm the suspected diagnosis?

For each scenario described below choose the *single* most likely diagnosis from the list of options. Each option may be used once, more than once or not at all.

1. Fluid movement

A. Osmotic pressure
B. Venous pressure
C. Osmolarity
D. Simple diffusion
E. Molarity
F. Co-transport
G. Facilitated diffusion
H. Osmolality
I. Oncotic pressure
J. Capillary pressure
K. Perfusion pressure
L. Active transport
M. Secondary active transport
N. Osmosis

Instruction: Match one of the terms given in the list above to the descriptions given below.

1. The force which tends to draw fluid back into a capillary. ☐
2. A measure of osmotic concentration of a solute independent of the concentration of other solutes. ☐
3. A process in which transport of one substance up its concentration gradient is coupled with the transport of a second substance down its concentration gradient. ☐
4. A process in which the flux of a solute is linearly related to concentration difference. ☐
5. The molar concentration of solute particles per litre of solution. ☐

2. Systemic and renal disease

A. Hyperosmotic dehydration
B. Glomerulonephritis
C. Essential hypertension
D. Diabetes mellitus
E. Renovascular hypertension
F. Hyposmotic dehydration
G. Urinary tract obstruction
H. Central diabetes insipidus
I. Oat cell carcinoma
J. Polydipsia
K. Nephrogenic diabetes insipidus

Instruction: Match one of the conditions listed above to the features given in the statements below.

1. Polyuria that responds to nasal application of antidiuretic hormone (ADH). ☐
2. Decrease in extracellular compartment volume, increase in intracellular compartment volume. ☐
3. Haematuria and proteinuria, oedema. ☐
4. Hypertension associated with increased plasma renin concentration. ☐
5. Hypertension of unknown cause. ☐

3. Diseases of the tubules and interstitium

A. Toxic acute tubular necrosis
B. Amyloidosis
C. Polycystic kidney disease
D. Urate nephropathy
E. Urinary tract infection
F. Sickle-cell disease nephropathy
G. Chronic pyelonephritis
H. Drug-induced tubulointerstitial nephritis
I. Goodpasture's syndrome
J. Ischaemic acute tubular necrosis
K. Acute pyelonephritis

Instruction: Match one of the renal diseases listed above to the case scenarios described below.

1. A 26-year-old woman who is 26 weeks pregnant, presents with a 2-day history of dysuria and increased frequency of micturition. On inspection of the urine sample, you notice it is cloudy. ☐
2. A 63-year-old man who has vesicoureteric reflux presents to the GP's surgery with a 3-day history of fever, general malaise and loin pain. He says he had also noticed that he suddenly needs to go to the toilet without warning. ☐
3. A 28-year-old male dies from a motorcycle accident in which he lost a lot of blood following trauma to his abdomen. Histological examination of the kidneys reveals infiltration of inflammatory cells and tubular cells, flattened and vacuolated tubular cells and interstitial oedema. ☐

4. A 70-year-old man with gout, now suffering from chronic kidney disease. ☐

5. A 30-year-old woman is found to have severe hypertension. Her mother reports she had bouts of 'undiagnosed' fever as a young child and wet the bed until age 12 following which she has always had nocturia. Urinalysis reveals the presence of protein. ☐

4. Signs in renal and urinary disease

A. Diabetic ketoacidosis
B. Bacterial endocarditis
C. Benign prostatic hyperplasia
D. Kidney transplant
E. Prostate carcinoma
F. Nephrotic syndrome
G. Hypertension
H. Carcinoma of the kidney
I. Stage 5 chronic kidney disease (CKD)
J. Renal osteodystrophy
K. Anaemia in CKD

Instruction: Match one of the renal diseases listed above to the clinical features given the statements below.

1. Large firm mass in the right iliac fossa with an overlying scar. ☐

2. Splinter haemorrhages present on the nails. ☐

3. Pale conjunctiva. ☐

4. Facial oedema. ☐

5. Prostate feels nodular on examination. ☐

5. Disorders involving the kidneys

A. Ectopic kidney
B. Membranoproliferative glomerulonephritis
C. Loop diuretics
D. IgA nephropathy (Berger's disease)
E. Renal artery stenosis
F. Nephrotic syndrome
G. Hypoplasia
H. Thiazide diuretics
I. Renal cell carcinoma
J. Hepatorenal syndrome

Instruction: Match one of the items listed above to the statements below.

1. A congenital abnormality of the kidney that predisposes to infection and stone formation. ☐

2. This is characterized by the presence of heavy proteinuria, hypoalbuminaemia and oedema, due to the glomerular capillary wall becoming excessively permeable to protein. ☐

3. The most common primary glomerular disease, causing recurrent haematuria, and in some cases, end-stage renal failure. ☐

4. A cause of secondary hypertension, due to poor renal perfusion and stimulation of renin secretion. ☐

5. These diuretics inhibit the Na^+/Cl^- co-transporter in the early distal tubule. They help reduce peripheral vascular resistance, and so are used to manage hypertension. ☐

6. Lower urinary tract abnormalities

A. Hydronephrosis
B. Hypertrophied bladder
C. Benign prostatic hypertrophy
D. Escherichia coli
E. Bladder diverticula
F. Hypotonic bladder
G. Candida albicans
H. Complete bifid ureters
I. Prostatitis
J. Hypospadias

Instruction: Match one of the lower urinary tract disorders listed above to the statements below.

1. The effect on the bladder if there is a lesion of afferent nerves from the bladder. ☐

2. A ureteric abnormality predisposing to infection, due to urinary reflux from the bladder. ☐

3. One of the most common pathogens causing cystitis. ☐

4. A 65-year-old male patient presenting with difficulty in starting to urinate, a poor stream of urine, post-micturition dribbling, frequency and nocturia is likely to have this condition. ☐

5. Obstruction at any point in the urinary tract causes increased pressure above the blockage. This is the term for the resultant dilatation of the renal pelvis and calyces. ☐

7. Blood and urine abnormalities in renal disease

A. Incontinence
B. Hyperkalaemia
C. Urinary tract infection
D. Hyperuricaemia
E. Conn's syndrome
F. 100 mg/L
G. Hypernatraemia
H. 300 mg/L
I. Uraemia
J. Syndrome of inappropriate ADH secretion (SIADH)

Instruction: Match one of the blood and urine abnormalities that commonly occur in renal diseases to the statements below.

1. Uncontrolled diabetes, incorrect fluid replacement, primary aldosteronism and fluid loss without replacement are all causes of this imbalance. ☐

2. A urine dipstick test can typically detect proteinuria, when the level of protein in the urine is greater than this value. ☐

3. This can result following treatment of lymphoma, leukaemia and in psoriasis. It can also be induced by drugs, such as thiazide diuretics. ☐

4. This is a cause of hypokalaemia (plasma [K$^+$] <3.5 mmol/L) resulting from increased renal losses. ☐

5. Risk factors include diabetes mellitus, impaired voiding, sexual intercourse, genitourinary malformations and impaired voiding due to obstruction. ☐

8. Symptoms and signs in renal and urinary disease

A. Chronic renal failure
B. Polycystic disease
C. Nephrotic syndrome
D. Benign nephrosclerosis
E. Ureteric obstruction
F. Abdominal bruit
G. Peritoneal dialysis
H. Bladder outflow obstruction
I. Haemodialysis
J. Nephritic syndrome

Instruction: Match one the conditions listed above to the statements below.

1. Microscopic haematuria, proteinuria and hypertension are typical features. ☐

2. Causes pain which typically radiates from the flank to the groin and iliac fossa (loin to groin). ☐

3. A patient presenting with dry, flaky, tanned-looking skin, scratch marks and bruises on his arms and abdomen. ☐

4. May suggest renal artery stenosis. ☐

5. A cause of irregular enlarged palpable kidneys. ☐

9. Renal function

A. Loop of Henle
B. Atrial natriuretic peptide
C. Proximal tubule
D. Water
E. Juxtaglomerular apparatus
F. Distal tubule
G. Urea
H. Bowman's capsule
I. Protein
J. Calcium

Instruction: Match one of the items listed above to the descriptions below.

1. The site of production of renin. ☐

2. In the glomerulus, the plasma is filtered through the capillary wall into this structure. ☐

3. 70% of filtered Na$^+$ is reabsorbed here by an Na$^+$/K$^+$ ATPase pump on the basolateral membrane. ☐

4. Antidiuretic hormone increases the permeability of the inner medullary collecting ducts to this substance. ☐

5. One of the actions of this substance is to reduce Na$^-$ reabsorption by the tubule, thus increasing Na$^+$ and water excretion by the kidney. ☐

10. Renal responses to systemic disorders

A. Afferent arterioles
B. β-blockers
C. NaCl and water retention
D. Metabolic alkalosis
E. Chronic pyelonephritis
F. Angiotensin-converting enzyme inhibitors
G. K$^+$ and water retention
H. Metabolic acidosis
I. Thiazide diuretics
J. Efferent arterioles

Instruction: Match one of the items listed above with the renal responses given below.

1. The kidney's response to hypoperfusion. ☐

2. A renal cause of secondary hypertension. ☐

3. In renal artery stenosis there is angiotensin II mediated vasoconstriction of these vessels to maintain glomerular capillary pressure. ☐

4. Acute renal failure may be precipitated by giving this drug to patients with renal artery stenosis. ☐

5. In hypovolaemic shock, the acid–base balance is disturbed, because Na$^+$ is retained, and is involved in the co-transport of H$^+$, K$^+$ and Cl$^-$. Cl$^-$ is reabsorbed in equal quantities, but there is increased H$^+$ and K$^+$ secretion, resulting in this state. ☐

Chapter 1 Basic principles

1. a. False ICF accounts for two-thirds TBW.
   b. True   Sodium is the major cation in ECF.
   c. True   Together, this accounts for one-third of TBW.
   d. True   These are both found in low concentrations in intracellular fluid.
   e. False Inulin is used to estimate glomerular filtration rate.

2. a. False Distilled water is a hypotonic solution, which draws water out of cells.
   b. False Water accompanies NaCl excretion in subject B; subject A has no extra NaCl, so free water clearance is higher.
   c. False Isotonic solutions have the same concentration as plasma.
   d. True   Subject B excretes extra NaCl, which increases urine osmolarity.
   e. False This is not altered.

3. a. False Hydrostatic pressure at the arterial end is 32 mmHg.
   b. False Oncotic pressure is constant due to the presence of plasma proteins.
   c. True   It is also determined by arteriole resistance and venous blood pressure.
   d. False They are impermeable and maintain a constant oncotic pressure.
   e. False Fluid returns at the venous end due to capillary oncotic pressure outweighing hydrostatic pressure.

4. a. False There is only 4 mmol/L Cl^- in the ICF compared with 103 mmol/L in the plasma.
   b. False There are proteins in the plasma, which makes up part of the ECF.
   c. False K^+ is predominantly an intracellular cation (150 mmol/L).
   d. False Transcellular fluid exists in body cavities such as in joints or in the central nervous system.
   e. True   The majority of our body weight is water within our cells.

5. a. True   This is measured using isotopes of water as markers.
   b. False This is a combination of plasma and erythrocyte volume.
   c. True   This can be measured using radiolabelled albumin.
   d. False This is the difference between total body water and extracellular fluid.
   e. False ISF = extracellular fluid − plasma volume.

6. a. False Daily losses through lung and skin are about 800 mL.
   b. True   Less is absorbed in the gut.
   c. True   Minimum water loss from urine, skin, lungs and faeces is about 1200 mL per day.
   d. False Water intake and output should be in balance.
   e. False About 400 mL of water per day is derived from metabolism.

7. a. True   Plasma osmolality is tightly controlled between 285 mOsmol/kg H_2O and 295 mOsmol/kg H_2O.
   b. False They are located in the anterior hypothalamus.
   c. True   Osmoreceptors monitor plasma osmolality in the internal carotid artery.
   d. False Non-osmotic stimuli including pain, nausea and pregnancy can stimulate ADH release.
   e. True   ADH reduces water loss in urine.

Chapter 2 Organization of the kidneys

8. a. True   The renal arteries branch off the abdominal aorta at level L1–20
   b. False Urine is drained from the kidney via the ureter, and from the bladder by the urethra.
   c. False The urinary tract is impermeable, only the nephrons within the kidney are permeable to water and solutes.
   d. False Renin is produced by the granular cells in the JGA.
   e. True   Bowman's capsule and the proximal tubule are in the cortex.

9. a. False Only 15% of nephrons have loops of Henle extending into the medulla.
   b. False It is water permeable.
   c. True   It is water impermeable.
   d. False The co-transporters are different.
   e. False ADH acts on the collecting duct.

10.
a. True The duodenum is an anterior relation.
b. False The inferior vena cava lies immediately lateral to the right kidney.
c. False It is lower due to the liver.
d. True The psoas lies posteriorly to both kidneys.
e. True The descending colon passes anteriorly.

Chapter 3 Renal function

11.
a. False It is usually between 8 mmol/L and 16 mmol/L.
b. False The difference between plasma anions and cations is unchanged.
c. False This increases the anion gap.
d. True Chronic uraemia leads to acidosis, which causes an increased anion gap.
e. True Excess metabolic production of acid increases the anion gap.

12.
a. False Diuretics cause hypokalaemia, which can be severe.
b. True Cholesterol levels can also rise.
c. True Hyperglycaemia can result.
d. False Calcium reabsorption is increased.
e. False They are used to treat hypertension and congestive cardiac failure.

13.
a. False Normal blood pH is 7.35–7.45.
b. True pH is low and HCO_3^- is reduced.
c. False Blood pH increases in alkalosis.
d. False pCO_2 is low as a result of hyperventilation stimulated by metabolic acidosis. In respiratory acidosis pCO_2 increases.
e. False Blood pH increases in alkalosis.

14.
a. True Renal tubule acidosis can cause hypokalaemia in the distal tubule.
b. True Flow rate in the collecting duct decreases lumen potassium, and thus increases potassium secretion.
c. True This is inversely proportional to potassium excretion.
d. True Potassium is excreted in association with H^+, so its excretion increases with a low blood pH.
e. True This increases potassium excretion.

15.
a. False The tuboglomerular feedback mechanism responds to changes in tubular fluid flow rate.
b. False The myogenic mechanism responds to changes in arterial pressure.
c. True The RBF determines how much fluid enters the glomerulus.

d. True Changes in distal NaCl concentrations are detected by the macular densa cells in the JGA, and influence changes in RBF by vasoconstriction of afferent arterioles.
e. False Feedback control is controlled by changes in tubular fluid flow rate and arterial pressure.

16.
a. False This causes alkalosis and an increase in blood pH.
b. False This causes a metabolic acidosis, with no change in pCO_2 and pO_2.
c. False This leads to vomiting, which causes a metabolic alkalosis.
d. True This acts as a respiratory centre depressant.
e. False This is associated with a respiratory alkalosis.

17.
a. False Glucose is transported by symport with Na^+ against its concentration gradient.
b. True If the plasma glucose concentration increases further, more glucose will be excreted in the urine.
c. False The amount filtered is proportional to the plasma phosphate concentration.
d. True In the presence of carbonic anhydrase, carbonic acid is converted to $H_2O + CO_2$, and to then re-form $HCO_3^- + H^+$ in the cell.
e. True Increased aldosterone levels result in increased K^+ secretion.

18.
a. False In order to reabsorb water in the collecting ducts, a hypertonic medulla is required.
b. True Active reabsorption of Na^+, K^+ and Cl^- reduces the osmolality of the tubular fluid.
c. False The thick ascending limb is impermeable to water.
d. True Due to increased osmolality in the medulla, NaCl diffuses down its concentration gradient into the tubular fluid.
e. False Maximum interstitial osmolality is 1400 Osmol/kg H_2O.

19.
a. False Aldosterone acts on the distal nephron to increase K^+ secretion.
b. False H^+ secretion is driven by active Na^+ reabsorption on the apical membrane.
c. False Strong acids are T_m-limited.
d. False Acidosis results in hyperkalaemia, thus decreasing K^+ secretion.
e. True As are strong organic acids and bases.

20.
a. True This is due to the negative charge of the filter.

b. False Filtration is driven by the hydrostatic pressure of the afferent arteriole.

c. True It prevents large molecules from being filtered.

d. False Poorly controlled diabetes may lead to either hyperfiltration acutely or glomerulosclerosis chronically.

e. False Protein should not be filtered at the glomerulus.

21. a. True Creatinine is freely filtered in the glomerulus.

b. False Clearance ratios compare the clearance of a substance with inulin.

c. False The eGFR is calculated using the MDRD equation.

d. True The eGFR is used in the clinical setting to measure renal function.

e. False Inulin is exogenous and is rarely used in clinical practice; creatinine is more widely used.

22. a. True Overbreathing increases CO_2 loss, which causes a respiratory alkalosis (pH increases).

b. False This is associated with a metabolic acidosis.

c. False This causes alkalosis due to loss of H^+ from vomiting.

d. False Blood gases are frequently normal.

e. False This causes a respiratory acidosis.

23. a. True Autoregulatory mechanisms maintain a constant RBF.

b. False PAH is used, but because it is freely filtered at the glomerulus and completely secreted by the proximal tubule.

c. False The tubuloglomerular mechanism also plays a vital role.

d. False RBF will fall.

e. True Adenosine is a vasoconstrictor and may reduce RBF, and nitric oxide is a vasodilator and has the opposite effect.

24. a. False This has a low pCO_2 and an elevated pH.

b. False pH falls in diabetic ketoacidosis, as a result of a metabolic acidosis.

c. False This does not reduce pO_2.

d. False Ingestion of alkali causes a metabolic alkalosis.

e. True This is associated with a gradual increase in pCO_2 and consequently there is a fall in pH.

25. a. False Osmoreceptors are located in the supraoptic and paraventricular areas of the anterior hypothalamus.

b. False ADH is regulated by serum osmolality. The sensation of thirst occurs at a higher serum osmolarity.

c. True V2 receptors are G-protein coupled, resulting in the phosphorylation of inactive aquaporins.

d. False Alcohol acts to inhibit ADH release.

e. False ADH increases collecting duct permeability via water channels called aquaporins.

26. a. False These are both symptoms of diabetes insipidus (and also of diabetes mellitus).

b. True This is failure of the kidneys to respond to circulating ADH.

c. False This may be a cause of failure of the kidneys to respond to ADH in nephrogenic diabetes insipidus.

d. True Such diseases include abscesses, stroke, tuberculosis and pneumonia.

e. True Na levels less than 125 mmol/L and low plasma osmolality (<260 mmol/L) are both signs.

27. a. True The kidneys receive 1.2 L/min of blood.

b. True This is the GFR.

c. True Substances over 70 kDa are too large to pass into the filtrate.

d. True This is driven by a sodium gradient, so sodium is reabsorbed simultaneously.

e. False Lipid-soluble substances can be reabsorbed.

28. a. False High levels of aldosterone negatively feedback to lower renin levels.

b. False Low plasma sodium stimulates renin secretion.

c. False Renin release is independent of potassium levels.

d. True A rise in ECF means an increase in blood pressure and reduces sympathetic stimulation of renin.

e. False Low Na^+ plasma levels lead to a fall in ECF volume and therefore stimulation of renin release.

29. a. False PTH is released from the parathyroid gland in response to falling plasma Ca^{2+}.

b. False PTH reduces phosphate reabsorption in the proximal tubule and increases urinary phosphate.

c. False Only ionized Ca^{2+} is filtered through the glomerulus which represents about 50% of total plasma Ca^{2+}.

d. True There is less H^+ to bind to protein so more Ca^{2+} can bind, leading to a decrease in ionized Ca^{2+}.

e. False   Renal calculi may be a sign of abnormally high calcium levels (hypercalcaemia).

30. a. True   Levels above 6.5 mmol/L may result in problems in cardiac conduction, and may lead to cardiac arrest and death.
    b. True   This leads to metabolic alkalosis due to H^+ loss, with compensation resulting in a loss of potassium from the plasma.
    c. False   ADH stimulates the secretion of K^+ by the collecting ducts by enhancing Na^+ absorption.
    d. False   Aldosterone increases potassium secretion, and reduces K^+ levels.
    e. True   Furosemide is a loop diuretic preventing reabsorption of K^+ in the thick ascending limb.

31. a. False   High blood protein levels do not alter the rate of filtration.
    b. False   This reduces urine flow, and GFR in an obstructed kidney falls.
    c. True   This increases renal perfusion pressure.
    d. False   This decreases glomerular capillary pressure and hence GFR falls.
    e. True   This increases glomerular capillary pressure and hence GFR increases.

32. a. False   ACE inhibitors may reduce erythropoietin.
    b. True   The erythropoietin gene is regulated by an oxygen-sensing mechanism.
    c. True   The tumour cells can produce erythropoietin.
    d. False   There are fewer cells available to secrete erythropoietin.
    e. False   This involves filtration of plasma proteins, with no change in erythropoietin secretion.

33. a. False   Creatinine is produced in muscle, and is higher in people with larger muscle bulk.
    b. False   Creatinine may be normal even when GFR has fallen by up to 50%.
    c. True   Tubular secretion of creatinine is reduced by certain drugs (cimetidine and trimethoprim).
    d. True   Muscle breakdown results in creatinine release.
    e. True   Creatinine clearance is used as a measure of GFR and creatinine may be used to estimate GFR (eGFR).

34. a. False   This causes metabolic alkalosis.
    b. True   Diabetes is a cause of ketoacidosis.
    c. True   There is failure to excrete acid.
    d. True   This is because of excess intake of acid.
    e. False   Aldosterone does not affect H^+/HCO_3^- metabolism.

Chapter 4 The kidneys in disease

35. a. False   It is more common in boys.
    b. True   The kidneys fail to develop and are also prone to infection.
    c. False   It is a lot lower, 1 in 800.
    d. True   Agenesis occurs if the collecting system fails to fuse with the nephrons.
    e. False   The ureters can be obstructed by neighbouring structures.

36. a. True   Up to 90% of childhood nephrotic syndrome.
    b. False   Podocyte fusion is seen only under the electron microscope.
    c. True   Any severe nephrotic illness is associated with an increased risk of infection.
    d. False   Treatment involves corticosteroids.
    e. False   Prognosis is better in children.

37. a. True   This may occur with patients requiring dialysis/transplantation.
    b. False   There is an autosomal recessive type which affects children or the fetus and may result in stillbirth.
    c. True   There are at least three PKD genes.
    d. False   Renal function tests are normal initially. Ultrasound or computed tomography (CT) is needed to diagnose PKD.
    e. False   The cysts can develop anywhere in the kidney.

38. a. False   This is usually a primary GN.
    b. False   It involves the alternative complement pathway.
    c. False   This is seen mainly in children and young adults.
    d. True   It can also present with haematuria or nephrotic/nephritic syndrome.
    e. True   This depends on the original cause of the GN.

39. a. False   It usually presents with haematuria or proteinuria.
    b. False   It is most common in France, Australia and Singapore.
    c. True   C3 and IgA is also deposited in the mesangium.
    d. False   There is no effective treatment.
    e. True   Hypertension is associated with more rapid progression.

40. a. True   This is characteristic of Goodpasture's syndrome.
    b. True   This can lead to acute renal failure.
    c. False   Patients develop acute renal failure.

d. True   This is more common in smokers.
e. False Patients require plasmapheresis.

41. a. True   This may be microscopic and is strongly indicative of glomerular damage.
    b. False It affects the glomerulus.
    c. True   Treatment of endocarditis will limit damage to the glomerulus.
    d. True   Indicates kidney involvement.
    e. True   These are deposited in the glomeruli.

42. a. False It is predominantly seen in children.
    b. True   It usually has an excellent prognosis in children.
    c. False It is immune mediated.
    d. True   Arthralgia is a common presenting feature
    e. True   One-third of patients have a glomerulonephritis histologically identical to IgA nephropathy.

43. a. True   Stasis occurs in the urinary tract due to the action of progesterone on smooth muscle.
    b. True   It is also mostly responsible for hospital-acquired UTIs.
    c. False A mid-stream specimen for culture and sensitivity is usually required to identify the specific organism.
    d. False NSAIDs can cause a T-cell mediated inflammation in the interstitium.
    e. False Diabetic people are more prone to UTIs especially when there is glycosuria.

44. a. False Occurs in IDDM and NIDDM (although as people with NIDDM are older many may die of cardiovascular disease before developing nephropathy).
    b. True   Nephropathy is a complication of long-standing, poorly controlled diabetes.
    c. True   Severe proteinuria causes nephrotic syndrome.
    d. True   Diabetes is the most common cause of end-stage renal disease.
    e. False It is characterized by microalbuminaemia in the early stages.

45. a. True   This occurs in 90% of cases.
    b. True   It occurs in a male to female ratio of 3:1.
    c. False It is malignant, so may metastasize.
    d. True   Increased erythropoietin levels can be detected and may cause polycythaemia.
    e. False Acquired cystic disease and Von Hippel–Lindau disease are other risk factors.

46. a. False Prevalence increases with age until 70, and they are more common in men.

b. True   Increases urinary solute concentration and predisposes to stone formation.
c. False Hypercalcaemia predisposes to stone formation.
d. False Thiazides reduce urinary calcium. Loop diuretics increase urinary calcium and may predispose to stone formation.
e. True   Excess glucocorticoids predispose to stone formation.

47. a. True   Hypertension develops due to increased circulating fluid volume (because of oliguria/anuria).
    b. True   This is due to fluid retention.
    c. True   GFR falls, so uraemic toxins accumulate.
    d. False This is not typical of an acute GN and may suggest haemolytic uraemic syndrome.
    e. False Haemorrhagic stroke may occur secondary to severe hypertension.

48. a. False The blood pressure will be low.
    b. True   This is caused by an increase in sympathetic tone.
    c. False Prostaglandins act to vasodilate vessels in the kidney to avoid excessive vasoconstriction.
    d. True   Aldosterone is released in response to increased renin levels in order to increase water retention.
    e. False Acid–base balance is commonly abnormal in shock.

49. a. True   Oedema is seen due to a fall in urine output and sodium and water retention.
    b. True   Oedema develops due to hypoproteinaemia and loss of intravascular oncotic pressure.
    c. False Loss of response to ADH causes polyuria and dehydration.
    d. False This does not impede urine production.
    e. False This is bladder infection, which does not affect urine output.

50. a. True   This accounts for at least 25% of all renal cases of hypertension cases.
    b. True   This is termed essential hypertension and is the most common type of hypertension.
    c. False A simple UTI will have little effect on blood pressure.
    d. False High levels of corticosteroids may cause hypertension, not low levels.
    e. True   These account for up to 75% renal causes of hypertension.

51. a. False ACE inhibitors act to inhibit the conversion of angiotensin I to angiotensin II.

b. True ACE inhibitors improve the outcome in heart failure.

c. False ACE inhibitors can cause developmental abnormalities or neonatal hypotension.

d. True Aldosterone release is inhibited.

e. True ACE inhibitors reduce proteinuria and delay progression in diabetic nephropathy.

52. a. False Loop diuretics are potent diuretics.

b. False Calcium excretion increases due to a lower positive lumen potential.

c. True This is the main site of action.

d. True Diuretics act to increase excretion of salt and water.

e. False This is seen with aldosterone antagonists.

53. a. False Typical indications include uraemia (GFR is 5–10 mL/min), urea >30 mmol/L, hyperkalaemia, acidosis and fluid overload.

b. True Haemodialysis, haemofiltration and peritoneal dialysis.

c. True It is constructed surgically, usually by joining the radial artery and cephalic vein.

d. False Complications include peritonitis.

e. False Complications include hypotension, infection and haemolysis.

54. a. False It is a treatment for end-stage chronic kidney disease.

b. False Like all transplants it has a risk of rejection.

c. False It is placed in the iliac fossa, and the donor renal vessels are anastomosed onto the iliac blood vessels.

d. True This is to minimize the chance of rejection.

e. True 1-year graft survival is 80% for cadaver and 90% for living related.

55. a. False Like furosemide, they can be used as a diuretic.

b. False They inhibit bicarbonate reabsorption.

c. True By reducing basic bicarbonate, metabolic acidosis can occur.

d. False They are weak diuretics.

e. False Their principal use is in glaucoma.

56. a. False This has equal sex incidence.

b. True It is commonly associated with giant cell arteritis.

c. True It is a systemic disorder.

d. True In comparison, microscopic PAN affects the small arteries of the body.

e. True PAN is a necrotizing vasculitis.

57. a. False This usually presents in children under 10 years old.

b. True Approximately 5% are bilateral.

c. False Lung metastases are common.

d. True Haematuria, pain or fever are also common.

e. True Treatment involves nephrectomy and chemotherapy.

58. a. False There is bilateral renal agenesis.

b. True This presents with respiratory distress at birth.

c. False Potter's syndrome is associated with oligohydramnios.

d. True The baby might be stillborn.

e. True These are characteristic features.

59. a. False Vesicoureteric reflux can be congenital or acquired.

b. True This is usually congenital.

c. True It frequently resolves with age.

d. True This is the result of chronic pyelonephritis and scarring with most damage being done in early childhood.

e. False Micturating cystourethrogram is used to show retrograde urine flow up the ureters while voiding.

60. a. False It most commonly affects 40–50-year-olds.

b. True It usually affects the kidneys, nose and upper respiratory tract.

c. False It is not inherited.

d. False This is characteristic of Henoch–Schönlein purpura.

e. True Treatment must be started as early as possible.

61. a. True No aldosterone is secreted, so sodium reabsorption is limited.

b. False Sodium and water is lost, so the ECF volume is depleted.

c. True There is volume depletion without a fall in the number of red blood cells, so the haematocrit increases.

d. True Exogenous corticosteroids suppress endogenous steroid production from the adrenal cortex.

e. False A decrease in aldosterone reduces potassium excretion causing hyperkalaemia.

62. a. True Acute renal impairment is usually associated with a fall in urine production.

b. False Renal impairment in nephritic syndrome is usually associated with salt and water retention and thus blood pressure increases.

c. True   This is due to glomerular injury.

d. False   Serum urea and creatinine may be normal or elevated.

e. True   This is post-streptococcal glomerular nephritis.

Chapter 5 The lower urinary tract

63. a. False   It is fixed by the puboprostatic and lateral vesical ligament.

b. False   This is under voluntary control and allows us to control our desire to void.

c. False   The prostate lies inferior to the bladder.

d. True   Parasympathetic stimulation results in relaxation and voiding whereas sympathetic stimulation has the opposite effect.

e. False   Supply is from the superior and inferior vesical branches of the internal iliac artery.

64. a. False   The incidence of BPH increases with age.

b. True   In comparison, prostate cancer is associated with tumours in the lateral lobes.

c. True   Surgery relieves the bladder outflow obstruction.

d. False   BPH is benign.

e. True   BPH causes obstruction and incomplete voiding which predisposes to UTI.

65. a. False   TCC is a malignant tumour.

b. True   This is a risk factor for TCC.

c. False   Squamous cell carcinoma is associated with schistosomiasis, which is common in Egypt.

d. False   Haematuria is usually painless.

e. True   This is the classic location for bladder TCC.

66. a. True   Demyelination occurs on the nerves, and with a loss saltatory conduction, lack of control may develop.

b. True   This acts to prevent micturition.

c. False   This has no effect on the control of micturition.

d. False   This disturbs acid–base balance but not to a degree to upset micturition.

e. True   The posterior neural arches fail to develop, so part of the spinal cord is exposed.

67. a. False   There is a strong predisposition to infection.

b. False   Hypospadias is not very common, occurring in 1 in 400 male infants.

c. True   This is due to bladder extrusion.

d. False   Acquired hydroureters exist an develop in pregnancy and lower urinary tract obstruction.

e. False   They may cause obstruction, bladder distention and renal failure with vomiting and failure to thrive.

68. a. False   This may lodge in the ureter and cause obstruction.

b. False   Urethral valves and strictures narrow the urethra.

c. False   The gravid uterus may obstruct the ureters.

d. True   This has no effect on the urinary tract patency, just on the fluid in it.

e. False   This may cause external compression of the urethra or ureters.

69. a. False   This is rare in the UK, but is the most common fluke infection worldwide.

b. True   This is the most common presentation.

c. False   The pathogen settles in the bladder to lay eggs.

d. True   Schistosomiasis infection predisposes to cystitis.

e. False   Treatment involves praziquantel, given daily.

70. a. False   Women are more at risk between puberty and their late 50s.

b. True   Smooth muscle relaxation leads to ureteric reflux.

c. True   Glucose in the urine encourages bacterial growth.

d. True   Urine reflux exposes the kidney to any lower urinary tract infection.

e. True   Postoperative infection can develop.

71. a. False   Parasympathetic stimulation results in the voiding of urine.

b. False   This occurs last otherwise urine would just leak out.

c. False   Under parasympathetic innervation, the detrusor muscle must contract to force urine out.

d. True   It is under involuntary control.

e. True   This results in parasympathetic stimulation of nerves from the sacral plexus.

72. a. False   It is common in elderly men, occurring in 1 in 10 men over 70.

b. True   This is a triad of hesitancy; poor stream; dribbling postmicturition, frequency and nocturia.

c. False   The tumour may extend locally beyond the prostate, and form metastases.

d. False   Digital rectal examination of the prostate should be done first.

e. True   Survival in T_1 tumours is a lot higher than if there is metastatic or local spread.

73. a. True   Male length is 20 cm, female length is 4 cm.
    b. False   There are three parts: prostatic, membranous and spongy.
    c. False   This occurs only in men; lymphatic drainage in women is to the internal and external iliac lymph nodes.
    d. False   The opening of the female urethra is into the vestibule, just anterior to the opening of the vagina.
    e. False   It passes through the prostate.

74. a. True   Stones can be detected incidentally.
    b. True   This can be microscopic or macroscopic.
    c. True   Pain occurs as the urinary tract muscle contracts to expel the stone.
    d. True   Stones and obstruction promote the growth of organisms in the urinary tract.
    e. True   As the stone enlarges, it can cause an obstruction.

75. a. False   This typically presents with microalbuminuria.
    b. True   Haematuria results from a necrotizing vasculitis, affecting glomerular capillaries.
    c. True   Haematuria results from trauma to the urinary tract from stones.
    d. False   This usually presents with proteinuria or nephrotic syndrome.
    e. False   This can result in haemoglobinuria.

76. a. False   They can be found in normal urine.
    b. False   The presence of any red cell casts is pathological.
    c. True   This suggests inflammatory response within the kidney to infection.
    d. True   Acute tubular necrosis results in tubular cell death and shedding into the tubular lumen.
    e. False   They indicate the nephritic syndrome.

Chapter 6 Common presentations of renal disease

77. a. False   These cause obstruction to urinary flow, and pain and haematuria.
    b. False   This is a structural abnormality of the lower urinary tract.
    c. True   This is one of the most common causes of proteinuria.
    d. True   This may be a sign of diabetic nephropathy.

e. True   Malaria can cause secondary nephrotic syndrome.

78. a. False   Overproduction of uric acid can occur without clinical gout.
    b. True   High cell turnover is a cause of hyperuricaemia – xanthine oxidase inhibitors are given prophylactically.
    c. True   Diuretics may cause hyperuricaemia.
    d. True   This suggests formation of urate stones, which are radiolucent.
    e. False   Hyperuricaemia refers to urate levels in the blood.

79. a. True   This may occur in uncontrolled diabetes where hyperglycaemia leads to an osmotic diuresis.
    b. False   There can be normal, high or low ECF volume in hyponatraemia.
    c. False   Conn's syndrome lowers K^+ levels.
    d. False   Too much insulin may cause a hypokalaemia by causing K^+ to move intracellularly.
    e. True   Acidosis results in hyperkalaemia whereas alkalosis has the opposite effect.

80. a. True   This is a systemic vasculitis with renal manifestations including a rapidly progressive glomerulonephritis.
    b. True   It is usually reversible but up to 5% will be irreversible as a result of permanent structural damage having occurred at the time of diagnosis.
    c. False   Dipsticks may be negative in acute tubular necrosis, the commonest cause of acute renal failure.
    d. True   NSAIDs cause a predictable fall in renal blood flow by inhibiting vasodilator prostaglandin production and can also cause acute interstitial nephritis in some patients.
    e. False   This has not been shown to improve the outcome of acute renal failure.

81. a. True   This is a non-steroidal drug. It can also cause minimal change glomerulonephritis.
    b. False   This does not affect renal function.
    c. True   An acute allergic reaction to the contrast can lead to renal failure.
    d. True   This is an ACE inhibitor and can cause a fall in GFR especially when there is renal artery stenosis.
    e. True   This is an antifungal drug, which can cause toxin-induced interstitial nephritis.

82. a. False   It can be seen in Reiter's, or as a result of irritation, phimosis and urethral carbuncles.

b. False   Smears and swabs for microscopy and culture are very important.

c. True   A triad of urethritis, conjunctivitis and polyarthritis.

d. False   Secretions may be cloudy and bloody.

e. True   Chlamydia and gonorrhoea are common sexually transmitted diseases which can cause a urethral discharge.

83. a. True   Urine production falls because glomerular filtration falls and there are fewer functioning nephrons.

b. True   As long as the initiating cause is promptly and effectively treated, acute tubular necrosis usually heals with supportive treatment.

c. False   Acute tubular necrosis causes hyperkalaemia which can be life-threatening.

d. True   Circulatory collapse secondary to sepsis is one of the major causes of acute tubular necrosis.

e. False   Acute tubular necrosis is an acute event and kidney size is typically normal.

84. a. True   This causes a membranous nephropathy, and the nephrotic syndrome.

b. True   This also causes a membranous nephropathy.

c. False   This does not cause proteinuria.

d. True   This is an ACE inhibitor, which can cause proteinuria.

e. False   This does not alter glomerular function.

85. a. False   They usually present with colicky type pain located to one quadrant of the abdomen.

b. True   Increased levels of plasma calcium increase urinary calcium and the risk of stone formation.

c. True   Patients with gout have high levels of urate which can also cause calculi.

d. False   Hyperparathyroidism can cause calculi by increasing plasma calcium concentrations.

e. False   High fluid intake will decrease the risk of further stone formation. Thiazide diuretics decrease hypercalcuria, and allopurinol will reduce uric acid levels.

86. a. True   Multiparous women may have weaker pelvic floor muscles.

b. True   These especially cause urge incontinence. Such examples are stroke, Parkinson's and Alzheimer's.

c. False   Overflow incontinence is associated with chronic urine retention.

d. False   A child may acquire a bedwetting problem called secondary nocturnal enuresis.

e. True   Before starting invasive procedures it is important to rule out a UTI.

87. a. True   Abnormal ureteric entry into the bladder causes reflux during voiding.

b. True   Excess glucose encourages bacterial growth.

c. True   In premenopausal women oestrogen stimulates vaginal secretions, which are bactericidal.

d. True   Chronic urinary retention and urinary stasis predispose to infection.

e. True   Examples include acquired or congenital urinary tract obstruction.

88. a. True   Intercourse can introduce bacteria into the bladder. Voiding flushes them out and helps prevent UTI.

b. True   This removes pathogens, preventing their accumulation in the urinary tract and avoids urinary stasis.

c. True   Glycosuria encourages bacterial growth in the urine.

d. True   A high fluid intake prevents a concentrated urine, thus reducing the risk of infection.

e. False   Immunosuppressants predispose to UTIs.

89. a. True   There is also subepithelial deposition of immune complexes.

b. False   It is more common in males.

c. True   A proliferative glomerulonephritis indistinguishable from IgA nephropathy is typically seen in Henoch-Schönlein purpura.

d. False   This is a chronic disease, with gradual onset.

e. False   Drug treatments include corticosteroids, ciclosporin and cyclophosphamide.

90. a. False   This requires antibiotic treatment.

b. True   This is a systemic vasculitis, effectively treated with steroids.

c. True   This is a connective tissue disorder, which requires steroid treatment.

d. False   This requires antibiotic treatment.

e. True   This is a systemic vasculitis.

Chapter 7 History and examination

91. a. True   High blood pressure can lead to chronic renal damage (nephrosclerosis).

b. True   Haematuria may indicate renal disease, but also has extrarenal causes.

c. True   A streptococcal infection may trigger a postinfective glomerulonephritis.

d. True To determine if the patient has been in specific areas which are associated with certain infections.

e. True A first-degree relative with diabetes increases the risk of acquiring the disease, which can lead to kidney damage if poorly controlled.

92. a. False Discoloration of the nails may indicate chronic kidney disease or nephrotic syndrome.

b. True This is due to a decrease in erythropoietin production, which causes anaemia.

c. False This can be caused by nephrotic syndrome, renal failure and acute GN.

d. True A dry cough is a side effect of treatment with ACE inhibitors.

e. False Difference in length of bones is seen in severe renal osteodystrophy.

93. a. False The patient should be flat.

b. False Inspection is always relevant to see scars, distension, discoloration and any obvious masses.

c. False Generally the patient should be examined from their right side.

d. False The signs are different; a kidney moves late with inspiration while the spleen moves early; you can feel above a kidney but not the spleen.

e. False Ascites also has cardiac and renal causes.

94. a. False A prostatic carcinoma feels nodular.

b. False Normal prostates are firm; a soft, tender and enlarged prostate indicates an infection.

c. False Assessment of the size and outline of the prostate is an essential part of the clinical examination.

d. True This is an intrusive examination and consent must be obtained.

e. True It also refers to its size.

Chapter 8 Investigation and imaging

95. a. False KUB specifies a complete view of the upper and lower urinary tract.

b. False 10% of stones are not visible on X-rays.

c. True This is the investigation of choice although other less invasive techniques can be used.

d. True Magnetic resonance imaging (MRI) can also be used.

e. False Contrast is injected into the renal artery.

96. a. True It can be used to differentiate between tumours and cysts.

b. False Ultrasound can only define size and anatomical abnormalities of the kidneys.

c. False Ultrasound can identify the pelvicalyceal system but the ureter is only seen if dilated.

d. True Ultrasound (transrectal) is the method of choice.

e. False Ultrasound may demonstrate obstruction to the urinary tract but will be normal in many causes of acute renal failure.

97. a. False Nitrites indicate a sign of infection.

b. True This is a quick assessment of urine that can be carried out at the bedside.

c. True Ketones suggest a ketoacidosis in diabetes mellitus but can be seen in starvation.

d. True Intake of beetroot or red food colourings can cause this.

e. False Glycosuria may have renal causes.

98. a. False Creatinine levels may be normal with up to 50% reduction in renal function. GFR accurately measures renal function.

b. False A raised PSA can also be explained by benign prostatic hyperplasia and acute prostatitis.

c. True Hypercalcaemia results in hypercalcuria and hence formation of calculi.

d. True It may be increased in infection, vasculitis or renal cell carcinoma.

e. False It is the opposite! This indicates a metabolic alkalosis.

99. a. True It is also used in the diagnosis of systemic diseases that affect the kidney.

b. False The needle is inserted posteriorly.

c. False Usually ultrasound guidance is used.

d. True This makes the procedure technically difficult.

e. False Bleeding is the main complication.

100. a. True These are pathogenic of active glomerular bleeding.

b. False Smooth, brown and soft crystals suggest uric acid containing stones.

c. False Bacteria are found in the urine only when there is an infection.

d. True Clots may indicate a carcinoma of the bladder or kidney.

e. True Bacteria and inflammatory cells can be identified on urine microscopy.

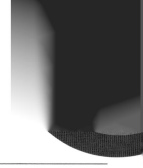

1. Body fluids can be divided into intracellular fluid (ICF), the fluid within the cells, and extracellular fluid (ECF), any other fluid that is outside the cells. In a 70 kg man, the ECF makes up around 20% of the total body weight and the ICF makes up 40%. One-third of the total body water is ECF and two-thirds is ICF. The ECF can be divided further into plasma, the fluid within the vascular system; interstitial fluid (ISF), the fluid outside the vascular system separated by the capillary endothelium; and transcellular fluid (TCF), fluid separated from the plasma by the capillary endothelium and an additional epithelial layer that has specialized functions.

2. The kidneys receive 20–25% of the total cardiac output (1.2 L/min). The blood enters the kidney via the right and left renal arteries. These branch to form about five interlobar arteries, which divide to form the arcuate arteries located at the junction between the cortex and medulla. The interlobular arteries are perpendicular to the arcuate arteries and pass through the cortex dividing up to form the afferent arterioles, which supply the glomerular capillaries. The efferent arterioles drain blood from the glomerular capillaries acting as portal vessels (i.e. carrying blood from one capillary network to another). In the outer two-thirds of the cortex the efferent arterioles form a network of peritubular capillaries that supply all the cortical parts of the nephron. In the inner third of the cortex the capillaries go on to follow a hairpin course adjacent to the loops of Henle and the collecting ducts down into the medulla. These vessels are known as the vasa recta. The vasa recta and the peritubular capillaries drain into the left and right renal veins and then into the inferior vena cava. (Figure 2.7 shows the microcirculation of the kidney.)

3. Proteins are very large negatively charged molecules that are unable to diffuse across membranes. If proteins are only present on one side of the membrane, they act to attract positive ions (cations) from the other side. Cations, therefore, diffuse across the membrane to maintain electrical neutrality. This means that one side will contain a greater number of ions. This results in a greater osmotic pressure on that side, which encourages the entry of water unless the pressure difference is balanced by hydrostatic pressure on the other side. Thus, according to this effect, there should be more ions inside the cell than outside. This is balanced by the presence of a Na^+/K^+ pump on the cell membrane, which pumps three Na^+ out of the cell in return for two K^+. This process requires energy in the form of ATP and results in a resting potential of -70 mV across the cell membrane.

4. Answers (refer to Chapters 4 and 5 for a detailed explanation) should include two of the following:
   - Double and bifid ureters
   - Uteropelvic obstruction
   - Ureteral or bladder diverticula
   - Hydroureters
   - Bladder exstrophy
   - Urethral valves
   - Horseshoe kidney
   - Pelvic kidney.

5. The nephron is the functional unit of the kidney in which molecules are filtered and reabsorbed. It consists of two parts; a renal corpuscle which contains the glomerulus and Bowman's capsule, and the tubule which has several different parts.
   The glomerulus is a network of capillaries, surrounded by Bowman's capsule – the very beginning of the renal tubule. The tubule then elongates within the cortex to form the proximal tubule. This is 15 mm long and is composed of a single layer of cuboidal cells in which their luminal edge is made up of millions of microvilli. The first part of the proximal tubule is convoluted and is named the pars convoluta, the second part is straight called the pars recta. The pars recta leads on to the first part of the loop of Henle, in the medulla. The loop of Henle constitutes a thin descending limb which descends into the inner medulla to form a hairpin loop which then ascends as a thin ascending limb. This limb thickens in the outer medulla to form the thick ascending limb. The thick ascending limb ascends into the cortex to form the distal convoluted tubule, ending in the collecting ducts in the medulla. The collecting ducts are 20 mm long, and drain urine at the apices of the renal pyramids into the renal pelvis.

6. Renal blood flow (RBF) and glomerular filtration rate (GFR) remain constant over a wide range of systemic blood pressure due to autoregulation. There are two mechanisms involved: the myogenic mechanism and the tubuloglomerular feedback mechanism.
   The myogenic mechanism involves reflex vasoconstriction in the afferent and efferent arterioles in response to stretch in their walls. If there is an increase in pressure in the afferent arteriole, stretch receptors are stimulated resulting in contraction of the smooth muscle. This vasoconstriction prevents the transmission of an increase in blood pressure to the glomerular capillary and thus maintains normal glomerular capillary pressure. The efferent arteriole contracts in response to a falling blood pressure, and acts to increase GFR and RBF.

The tubuloglomerular feedback mechanism involves the monitoring of NaCl flow and concentration at the macula densa. If the GFR rises, the tubular flow rate increases, less NaCl is reabsorbed and a greater concentration is detected at the macula densa. This triggers the juxtaglomerular apparatus to release vasoconstrictors to lower the RBF and GFR. (The main vasoconstrictors and vasodilators are summarized in Figure 3.5.)

---

7. Antidiuretic hormone (ADH) is released from the posterior pituitary in response to an increase in ECF osmolality. ADH in the blood binds to V2 receptors on the basolateral membrane of the collecting tubule cells. These receptors are G-protein bound receptors, which on stimulation cause the cleaving of ATP to form cyclic AMP (cAMP). cAMP then acts to activate a previously inactive protein kinase (PKA). Now, the active PKA causes phosphorylation and activation of the vesicles containing aquaporin 2 (AQP2) channels. The result is a fusion of the vesicles and AQP2 channels with the luminal membrane. This makes the collecting duct much more permeable to water with a resultant increase in water reabsorption from the collecting duct and the production of a more concentrated urine.

---

8. Renin is an enzyme that is stored in the juxtaglomerular apparatus (JGA) in the kidneys, and it is responsible for increasing the extracellular fluid (ECF) volume and body Na^+ when there is hypovolaemia. Its release is triggered by several mechanisms:

- First, a fall in ECF volume results in a fall in blood pressure. This is detected by baroreceptors in the carotid arteries and causes increased sympathetic activity. The granular cells of the JGA receive sympathetic innervation, and so on stimulation, release renin.
- Second, a fall in ECF reduces the blood pressure in the kidneys. This decrease is felt as a fall in wall tension at the JGA, and so the granular cells release renin in order to restore blood pressure.
- Third, if less Na^+ arrives at the macula densa, prostaglandins are released to act on the granular cells to produce renin.

Renin exerts its action through the renin–angiotensin–aldosterone system (Fig. 3.15). Renin acts to convert angiotensinogen to angiotensin I. The angiotensin-converting enzyme (ACE) converts angiotensin I to angiotensin II, a powerful vasoconstrictor responsible for increasing blood pressure to normal levels. Angiotensin II also acts on the adrenal cortex, stimulating the release of aldosterone. Aldosterone increases Na^+ reabsorption and thus increases water retention. This results in an increase in ECF volume, back to normal level.

---

9. The normal range for plasma glucose is 2.5–5.5 mmol. About 0.2–0.5 mmol of glucose is filtered every minute if the plasma concentration is normal. Any increase in the plasma glucose concentration results in a proportional increase in the amount of glucose filtered. Virtually all the filtered glucose is reabsorbed in the proximal tubule unless the filtered glucose exceeds the resorptive capacity of the cells.

Glucose is transported into the proximal tubular cells against its concentration gradient by active transport (a symport). Glucose reabsorption is driven by energy released from the transport of sodium down its electrochemical gradient as the Na^+/K^+ ATPase pump on the basolateral membrane maintains a low sodium concentration and negative potential within the cell. Figure 2.21 shows glucose transport in cells of the pars convoluta. The transport ratio is 1:1 sodium:glucose in the pars convoluta and 2:1 sodium:glucose in the pars recta.

All the nephrons have different thresholds for glucose reabsorption (nephron heterogeneity). T_m is the maximum tubular resorptive capacity for a solute (i.e. the point of saturation for the carriers) and this value can be calculated for glucose. The number of Na^+/glucose carrier molecules is limited and so glucose reabsorption is T_m limited. Figure 2.22 shows the relationship between glucose reabsorption and excretion depending on the plasma concentration. The graph shows that the lowest renal threshold of glucose is at a plasma glucose of 10 mmol/L. At this level, filtered glucose will begin to be excreted in the urine (glycosuria). As plasma glucose concentration increases further (as can occur in uncontrolled diabetes mellitus) even the nephrons with highest resorptive capacity will allow glucose excretion and urinary glucose increases in parallel with plasma glucose. The T_m is reached at a plasma glucose concentration of 20 mmol/L.

In pregnancy the renal threshold for glucose is temporarily decreased and glucose can appear in the urine even when blood glucose is less than 10 mmol/L (renal glycosuria).

---

10. Calcium and phosphate concentrations in the plasma are inversely related. Parathyroid hormone (PTH) plays a major role in maintaining calcium and phosphate balance. PTH is released in response to a fall in plasma Ca^{2+}. It acts on the kidney in the following ways:

- Increases Ca^{2+} reabsorption in the distal tubules
- Decreases phosphate reabsorption in proximal tubule and thus increases urinary excretion of phosphate
- Forms active vitamin D which increases Ca^{2+} absorption in the gut, and increases bone resorption. (Vitamin D is acquired through food or by the action of ultraviolet light on certain provitamins in the skin.)

PTH increases plasma Ca^{2+} further more by increasing bone resorption, which releases Ca^{2+} into the blood. Calcitonin is a peptide produced in the thyroid gland which also controls calcium levels to a small degree. It acts to reduce Ca^{2+} from bone, causing a decrease in plasma Ca^{2+} levels.

11. The answer should include brief information about the following conditions:
   - Immune-complex-mediated (systemic lupus erythematosus (SLE), Henoch–Schönlein purpura (HSP) and bacterial endocarditis)
   - Pauci-immune vasculitis (polyarteritis nodosa, Wegener's granulomatosis)
   - Metabolic (diabetes, amyloidosis).

12. Nodular and diffuse glomerulosclerosis, arteriolar lesions, and exudative lesions such as the fibrin cap are all renal manifestations of diabetes mellitus. On electron microscopy there is an increase in the thickness of the glomerular basement membrane and an increase in mesangial matrix with two morphological patterns: (i) nodular glomerulosclerosis (Kimmelstiel–Wilson nodules) – nodular accumulations of mesangial matrix material; and (ii) diffuse glomerulosclerosis – diffusely increased areas of mesangial matrix.

    The onset of diabetic nephropathy is clinically manifested by the development of microalbuminuria followed by overt proteinuria, which can reach the nephrotic range. There is then a progressive fall in glomerular filtration rate (GFR), which is commonly associated with hypertension. Diabetic nephropathy is usually associated with diabetic complications in other organs (especially retinopathy). Diabetes mellitus has usually been present for over 20 years before end-stage renal failure develops. In developed countries, diabetic nephropathy is the most common reason for needing dialysis or a kidney transplant.

    Pyelonephritis is a common complication in patients with diabetes mellitus and can cause renal papillary necrosis.

13. Refer to Figure 5.15. The T staging describes tumour invasion of the tissue, N staging describes the degree of spread to the lymph nodes and M staging describes the presence or absence of metastases. Answers should include the following:
    a. T1 describes invasion into the lamina propria.
       T2 describes invasion through the lamina propria into the superficial muscularis propria.
       T3 describes invasion into the deep muscularis propria and perivesical fat.
       T4 describes invasion through all the above mentioned and into adjacent structures.
    b. N1 describes local node involvement.
       N2 describes distant nodes below the diaphragm.
       N3 describes distant nodes on both sides of the diaphragm.
    c. M0 means the absence of metastases.
       M1 describes the presence of metastases.

14. In 2–5% of patients with hypertension, the hypertension is secondary to renal artery stenosis (RAS) in one or both renal arteries. The stenoses is usually due to atheromatous plaques (90%+) within the renal artery wall or rarely fibromuscular dysplasia. This results in excessive renin secretion by the affected kidney because there is renal hypoperfusion and this is interpreted as a fall in body fluid volume. There is also a small degree of renal ischaemia. Treatment to dilate the stenosis (angioplasty) or corrective surgery, may aid blood pressure control and preserve renal function in some cases. If the blood pressure is left uncontrolled the contralateral kidney might become damaged by hypertension. People with RAS rely on constriction of the efferent renal arteriole to maintain pressures for glomerular filtration on the affected side. Angiotensin II is the main agent responsible for constriction of these vessels. Angiotensin-converting enzyme inhibitors cause a decrease in angiotensin II and will dramatically decrease glomerular capillary pressure within the kidney, resulting in acute renal failure.

15. Potassium levels may be either too high (hyperkalaemia) or too low (hypokalaemia). Hypokalaemia has many causes and can result form renal losses, extrarenal losses and transcellular shifts. Renal losses are caused by the use of diuretics and excess mineralocorticoids (Conn's syndrome). Extrarenal losses can be due to diarrhoea and severe vomiting. Potassium is the main intracellular cation, and is actively maintained within the cells. This may be disrupted when there are transcellular shifts such as in metabolic alkalosis or too much insulin administration in diabetes. Hypokalaemia is asymptomatic until potassium concentration falls below 2–2.5 mmol/L. The low potassium concentration hyperpolarizes nerve and muscle cells. This means that cells are less sensitive to depolarization, so fewer action potentials are generated, resulting in paralysis. The clinical effects are muscle weakness and cramps, impaired liver glycogen formation, impaired antidiuretic hormone action and metabolic alkalosis due to an increase in intracellular H^+.

    Hyperkalaemia also has many different causes. Low aldosterone levels in adrenal insufficiency result in less K^+ being secreted into the tubular fluid and excreted in the urine, thus leading to an increase in plasma potassium. Potassium-sparing diuretics (spironolactone) also increase plasma potassium as do angiotensin-converting enzyme inhibitors by inhibiting the production of aldosterone. Hyperkalaemia may also occur in renal failure as renal potassium excretion is reduced. Metabolic acidosis can also result in abnormally high potassium because of increases in H^+ excretion in the urine. The effects of hyperkalaemia can be fatal. There is an increase in excitability of nerves and cells, meaning that the resting potential might be above the threshold potential. Fatal arrhythmias can occur when potassium levels are greater than 7 mmol/L. Treatment includes dextrose and insulin to drive potassium intracellularly, administration of calcium to stabilize cell membranes and correction of the underlying pathological cause. Dialysis may be required.

---

16. Prostatic hypertrophy results in incomplete emptying of the bladder. This may cause a number of lower urinary tract symptoms including poor stream, frequency, hesitancy, terminal dribbling and nocturia. Obstruction of urine flow is associated with compensatory hypertrophy of the bladder wall as a result of high pressures that develop within the bladder for voiding (Fig. 5.8). This may cause:

- Bands of thickened smooth muscle fibre cause trabeculation of the bladder wall
- Formation of diverticula on the external surface of the bladder
- Bladder dilation once the muscle becomes hypotonic
- Hydroureter formation resulting in reflux of urine up to the renal pelvis
- Bilateral hydronephrosis
- Urinary tract sepsis
- Stone formation
- Renal failure.

---

17. a. The bruits are a sign of vascular disease; they develop as a result of atheromatous narrowing in the blood vessels. The abdominal bruits suggest renal artery stenosis (RAS). The carotid bruit is the most likely origin for an embolus, which could have caused the stroke.

b. The likely diagnosis is hypertension and impaired renal function secondary to RAS. The patient also has hypercholesterolaemia, which predisposes to atherosclerosis and RAS.

c. Renal angiography is the investigation of choice and gives the potential to proceed to angioplasty – magnetic resonance angiography could also be used.

d. Patients with RAS have high circulating levels of angiotensin II, which acts to constrict efferent arterioles and maintain glomerular filtration rate (GFR). Angiotensin-converting enzyme inhibitors reduce angiotensin II and cause efferent arteriolar dilatation, and therefore cause an acute fall in GFR.

e. The patient does not require dialysis because renal function, although impaired, is still acceptable.

f. Management includes blood pressure control, treatment of cholesterol and antiplatelet agents (aspirin). Vascular 'risk factors' should be assessed and corrected where possible (smoking, weight loss, exercise) The RAS and carotid artery stenosis should be investigated. Treatment with angioplasty or surgery may be indicated depending on the severity. Renal function should be monitored regularly.

18. a. A digital rectal examination must be performed. This will confirm any prostatic enlargement, and help differentiate between benign prostatic hypertrophy ((BPH) feels smooth) and prostatic carcinoma (hard and irregular). Transrectal ultrasound scan (TRUS) will help define prostate size and outline, and, if necessary, guide a biopsy of the prostate to allow a histological diagnosis.

b. As stated above, the two most likely diagnoses in a male patient above the age of 40 are BPH and prostate cancer.

c. Prostatic cancer is associated with a rise in prostate-specific antigen (PSA). However, it should be noted that a normal PSA does not exclude prostate carcinoma and PSA may be slightly elevated in BPH.

19. a. The most likely diagnosis is nephrotic syndrome, of which the most common cause in children would be minimal change glomerulonephritis. It is more common in Asians, and in males.

b. Useful investigations include urine dipstick (gross proteinuria), quantification of proteinuria (>3 g/24 h) and measurement of serum albumin (<25 g/L) and cholesterol (elevated). Renal function tests (i.e. urea, creatinine, etc.) should also be measured. Autoantibody screen hepatitis B and C (and possibly human immunodeficiency virus (HIV)) should be checked looking for secondary causes of the nephritic syndrome (rare in this age group).

c. Treatment involves diuretics to relieve the oedema, salt and fluid restriction. Oral steroids (prednisolone) cause remission in the majority of cases of minimal change disease. In the acute phase if the nephrosis is severe, antibiotic prophylaxis because of the risk of sepsis and anticoagulation because of the risk of thrombosis may be required.

20. a. The most likely explanation for this presentation is a bladder calculus. As the bladder empties, the bladder wall contracts, forcing the stone against the bladder wall. This irritates the bladder lining, causing pain and bleeding.

b. The patient also has pain in his penis since this receives its sensory supply from the pudendal nerve (S1–S3) and the ilioinguinal nerve (L1–L2). The bladder is also innervated by these segments, so pain is referred to the penis. On lying down, the bladder stone rolls back, no longer irritating the trigone membrane. Consequently, the pain is alleviated.

c. The investigation of choice to confirm the presence of stones is an ultrasound. Alternatively, a kidney-ureter-bladder (KUB) radiograph can be ordered.

1. Fluid movement

1. I Oncotic pressure – mainly due to the presence of proteins.

2. H Osmolality – molar concentration of solute particles per kilogram of solvent.

3. M Secondary active transport – examples are symport and antiport.

4. D Simple diffusion – no energy is required in this process.

5. C Osmolarity – not to be confused with osmolality.

2. Systemic and renal disease

1. H Central diabetes insipidus – a problem with ADH production, rather than ADH resistance.

2. F Hyposmotic dehydration – more salt is lost than water, such as in adrenal insufficiency.

3. B Glomerular nephritis – the inflammation of the glomerulus makes the glomerular barrier 'leaky' and interferes with its ability to stop red cells and proteins being filtered.

4. E Renovascular hypertension – renin release leads to vasoconstriction through angiotensin II which raises blood pressure.

5. C Essential hypertension – the most common type of hypertension.

3. Diseases of the tubules and interstitium

1. E Urinary tract infection – common is pregnancy due to high levels of progesterone and smooth muscle relaxation.

2. K Acute pyelonephritis – the ascending infection causes the systemic signs.

3. J Ischaemic acute tubular necrosis – the blood loss following the trauma causes hypoperfusion and ischaemia.

4. D Urate nephropathy – high uric acid levels in gout may deposit in the kidney and lead to fibrosis and atrophy. Chronic renal impairment as a result of the use of non-steroidal anti-inflammatory drugs (NSAIDs), which are commonly taken for gout, is also a possibility.

5. G Chronic pyelonephritis – infection (usually in early childhood) results in chronic scarring and can lead to hypertension and chronic renal failure. This is a T-cell mediated inflammatory response.

4. Signs in renal and urinary disease

1. D Kidney transplant – usually transplanted in this position, with its vessels anastomosed to the iliac vessels.

2. B Bacterial endocarditis – this causes a systemic vasculitis.

3. K Anaemia in CKD – there is no iron deficiency here, just a decrease in erythropoietin.

4. F Nephrotic syndrome – the loss of protein in the urine corrupts the body's mechanism of drawing fluid back into the blood.

5. E Prostate carcinoma – it is usually hard, irregular and nodular.

5. Disorders involving the kidneys

1. A Ectopic kidney – the kidney does not ascend fully into the abdomen, so the ureters can be obstructed by neighbouring structures

2. F Nephrotic syndrome – glomerular basement membrane damage and increase in pore size allows greater permeability to albumin.

3. D IgA nephropathy – this typically affects young men after an upper respiratory tract infection. IgA deposition is seen in the mesangium.

4. E Renal artery stenosis – there are two types; atherosclerosis, which is common; and fibromuscular dysplasia, which is rare.

5. H Thiazide diuretics – renal side effects include hypokalaemic metabolic alkalosis, hyperglycaemia, hyperlipidaemia and hyperuricaemia.

6. Lower urinary tract abnormalities

1. F Hypotonic bladder – lesion prevents reflex contraction of the bladder, so it becomes distended and thin walled.

2. H Complete bifid ureters – this results from early splitting of the ureteric bud or the development of two buds. One of the ureters inserts abnormally into the bladder allowing reflux of urine

3. D *Escherichia coli* – *Proteus* species and *Enterobacter* are other common pathogens. *Candida albicans* causes cystitis in patients on long-term antibiotics.

4. C Benign prostatic hypertrophy – enlargement of the prostate, which compresses the

prostatic urethra and the periurethral glands swell, affecting the bladder

5. A   Hydronephrosis – there is unilateral or bilateral dilation of the renal tract above the obstruction.

7. Blood and urine abnormalities in renal disease

1. G   Hypernatraemia – serum sodium >140 mmol/L. In the conditions listed there is an increase in solute to water ratio in body fluids, increasing serum osmolality.

2. H   300 mg/L – microalbuminaemia is the presence of excess urinary albumin but in amounts insufficient to cause a positive dipstick analysis.

3. D   Hyperuricaemia – uric acid = 480 µmol/L for men, and = 390 µmol/L for women. It may cause gout.

4. E   Conn's syndrome – hypokalaemia can also be caused by transcellular shift, and by extrarenal losses due to, among other things, diarrhoea and vomiting.

5. C   Urinary tract infection – it can occur with or without leucocytes, caused by migration of bacteria up the urethra into the bladder, ureter and kidney

8. Symptoms and signs in renal and urinary disease

1. J   Nephritic syndrome – the signs and symptoms are decreased urine output, hypertension, oedema, haematuria, proteinuria and renal impairment.

2. E   Ureteric obstruction – acute obstruction to the ureter typically causes pain with this distribution.

3. A   Chronic renal failure – this can cause an increase in photosensitive pigment due to decreased clearance of porphyrins in the urine, and increased melanin secondary to increased melanocyte-stimulating hormone. Uraemia may also result in platelet dysfunction causing bruising.

4. F   Abdominal bruit – this is the noise caused by turbulent blood flow through the narrowed arteries.

5. B   Polycystic disease – multiple cysts develop in the kidneys from dilated tubules and Bowman's capsules.

9. Renal function

1. E   Juxtaglomerular apparatus – the tunica media in the wall of the afferent arteriole contains an area of granular cells, which secrete renin.

2. H   Bowman's capsule – the capsule is lined by a single layer of podocytes, which rest on the basement membrane.

3. C   Proximal tubule – the luminal edge of each tubule is made up of millions of microvilli, forming a dense brush border that increases the surface area.

4. G   Urea – ADH also regulates the movement of water out of the collecting ducts in the loop of Henle.

5. B   Atrial natriuretic peptide – it is produced by cardiac atrial cells in response to an increase in ECF volume.

10. Renal responses to systemic disorders

1. C   NaCl and water retention – CCF leads to a fall in CO, causing renal hypoperfusion.

2. E   Chronic pyelonephritis – Chronic glomerulonephritis and polycystic kidney disease are also causes.

3. J   Efferent arterioles – constriction of the efferent arteriole by angiotensin maintains glomerular capillary pressure and glomerular filtration rate.

4. F   Angiotensin-converting enzyme inhibitors – they are used to treat hypertension as they decrease the production of angiotensin II so decrease vasoconstriction.

5. D   Metabolic alkalosis – this is also known as contraction alkalosis. Hypokalaemia also occurs in hypovolaemic shock.

Acute renal failure A significant deterioration in renal function occurring over hours or days. Clinically, there may be no symptoms or signs, but oliguria (urine volume <400 mL/24 h) is common.

Agenesis A condition in which a part of the body (such as an organ or a tissue) does not completely develop or fails to develop at all.

Albumin A plasma protein synthesized by the liver, responsible for maintaining blood volume by its osmotic tendencies.

Anaplastic Characteristics of a cell (structure and orientation) that make it identifiable as a cancer cell and malignant.

Antidiuretic hormone (ADH) A hormone released from the posterior pituitary, which acts to increase water reabsorption from the collecting tubules.

Anuria No urine production.

Aquaporins Protein water channels, involved in the reabsorption of water in the collecting tubules.

Chronic kidney disease (CKD) The presence of structural and or functional alterations within the kidney. It may (but doesn't always) lead to irreversible loss of renal function which is termed chronic renal failure.

Countercurrent multiplier The process by which the loop of Henle and the vasa recta system maintain a hypertonic medulla to concentrate urine.

Creatinine A waste product of protein metabolism. It is excreted by the kidneys predominantly as a result of glomerular filtration.

Davenport diagram A diagram showing acid–base disturbances and their compensatory mechanisms.

Diabetes insipidus Failure of ADH secretion or action; neurogenic or nephrogenic.

Dorsiflexion Turning upwards of the foot or toes or of the hand or fingers.

Dysplasia Abnormality of development, alteration in size, shape and organization of adult cells.

Epispadias A congenital defect resulting in the urethral opening on the dorsum of the penis.

Erythropoiesis Process of erythrocyte production.

Glomerular filtration rate (GFR) The amount of filtrate that is produced from the blood flowing through the glomerulus per unit time.

Glycosuria The presence of glucose in the urine.

Gram's stain A stain for bacterial cells, used as a prime method of identification. Bacteria are divided into Gram −ve, those bacteria which lose the stain, and Gram +ve, those which retain the stain. These differences are based on variations in the structure of the cell walls of the different groups.

Haematocrit The percentage of red blood cells in total blood volume.

Haematuria The passage of blood in the urine. This may be seen by the naked eye (frank haematuria) or urine microscopy (microscopic haematuria).

Hydronephrosis Abnormal dilatation of a kidney; may occur secondary to acute ureteral obstruction (kidney stone).

Hydrostatic pressure The pressure of a fluid depending on arteriole blood pressure, resistance and venous blood pressure.

Intramural Being within the substance of the walls of an organ.

MDRD equation Equation used to calculate eGFR, which takes into account the serum creatinine level, age, sex and race of the patient.

Mesenchyme Embryonic tissue of mesodermal origin.

Nephrectomy The surgical removal of a kidney.

Oliguria Production of a diminished amount of urine in relation to the fluid intake (<400 mL/day).

Osmotic pressure The pressure of a fluid's osmotic effect due to the presence of plasma proteins and the imbalance of ions.

Osteodystrophy Defective bone formation.

p-Aminohippuric acid (PAH) An organic acid which is filtered and secreted in the tubules, used to measure renal blood flow.

Parenchyma The essential elements of an organ, used in anatomical nomenclature as a general term to designate the functional elements of an organ, as distinguished from its framework or stroma.

Percutaneous Performed through the skin.

Polycythaemia Increase in the haemoglobin content of the blood, either because of a reduction in plasma volume or an increase in red cell numbers.

Proteinuria The presence of protein in the urine. This may indicate damage to, or disease of, the kidneys.

Pyelitis Inflammation of the pelvis of the kidney.

Renin–angiotensin–aldosterone axis A molecular cascade stimulated in response to a falling extracellular fluid volume in order to maintain Na^+ balance.

Retroperitoneal Posterior peritoneum.

Sclerosis The development of fibrosis usually following inflammation (i.e. glomerulosclerosis).

SIADH Syndrome of inappropriate ADH secretion.

Tophi Pleural of tophus, a hard deposit of crystalline uric acid and its salts in the skin, cartilage or joints.

Uraemia The constellation of signs and symptoms that result from chronic renal failure.

Xiphisternum The posterior segment, or extremity, of the sternum.

Page numbers in italics refer to diagrams and flow charts.

A

abdomen examination 151–4, 176
abdominal aorta *4*, 15
absence of the kidney 65–6
acid phosphate 53, *54*
acid–base disturbances 54–8, *56*, 58, 187, 189
acidosis 31, 184, 190
   metabolic 54, 57, 171, 181, 184, 185, 195
   respiratory 54, 55–7
Acinetobacter 78
acquired cystic disease 68
active transport 7–8, 24–5, *26*, 179
acute renal failure (ARF) 126, 129–30, 175
acute tubular necrosis (ATN) 77–8, 175, 190, 191
adenocarcinoma 113
adenoma, cortical 83
adenosine 42, 43, 171, 185
adenosine diphosphate (ADP) 25
adenosine triphosphate (ATP) 7, 24–5, 194
adrenal glands *4*, *14*, 15, *15*, 19, 49, 84
adrenal steroids 47
adrenocortical insufficiency 173
afferent arterioles 17, 181, 193, 198
   action of atrial natriuretic peptide 51
   function of 16
   hydrostatic pressure of 185
   myogenic mechanism 24
   thrombotic microangiopathies 82–3
   vasoconstriction of 171, 184
   wall tension of 49
afferent nerves from the bladder, lesion of 103
agenesis of the kidney 65–6, 186
albumin 9, 23, 183
alcohol 46, 185
aldosterone 49–50, *50*
   action of atrial natriuretic peptide on 51
   function of 92
   hyperaldosteronism 89
   K^+ excretion 31, 32, 61, 170
   K^+ secretion 184, 185
   Na^+ transport 27, 188
   regulation of urine concentration 37
   renal artery stenosis 88
   renin levels 186, 187
   see also renin–angiotensin–aldosterone (RAA)
       system
alkaline phosphate 53, *54*

alkalosis
   metabolic 54, 57–8, 181, 184, 186, 192, 198
   respiratory 54, 57, 185
Alport's syndrome 69
alternative complement pathway, activation of *72*, 73
amino acids 27–8, 29–30
ammonia secretion 53–4, *55*, *56*
amphotericin 175
amyloidosis 76–7, 179
anaemia 20, 180, 197
analgesic abuse 80
anatomy of the kidneys 14, *14*
angiomyolipoma 83
angioplasty, therapeutic 161
angiotensin 19, 49
   see also renin–angiotensin–aldosterone (RAA)
       system
angiotensin-converting enzyme (ACE) 49, 194
angiotensin-converting enzyme (ACE) inhibitors 173
   action of 187–8
   chronic kidney disease 131
   congestive cardiac failure 86
   erythropoietin 186
   hypertension management 89–90, *90*, 198
   renal artery stenosis 177
   side effects of 192
angiotensinogen 49
anion gap 57, 129, 158, 170, 184
anions 7, *8*, 57, 184
antegrade pyelography 162–3
antidiuretic hormone (ADH) 171, 183, 185, 186, 194
   angiotensin II 49
   bedwetting 43
   concentration of urine 36
   diabetes insipidus 37, 197
   distal tubule 17
   hyperuricaemia 123
   kinins 51
   maintaining osmolality *44*, 44–7, *45*, *48*
   polyuria 179
   potassium secretion 61
   urea 31, 198
   urine concentration 37
   see also syndrome of inappropriate ADH secretion
       (SIADH)
antiglomerular basement membrane (anti-GBM)
      disease 72
antineutrophil cytoplasmic antibodies (ANCA) 77
antiport 25
aorta, abdominal *4*, 15